Denying AIDS

Seth C. Kalichman

Denying AIDS

Conspiracy Theories, Pseudoscience, and Human Tragedy

Foreword by Nicoli Nattrass

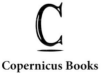

Copernicus Books

An Imprint of Springer Science+Business Media

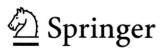 Springer

Visit the author's blog at http://denyingaids.blogspot.com/

Springer Science+Business Media, LLC © 2009

Published in the United States by Copernicus Books,
an imprint of Springer Science+Business Media.

Copernicus Books
Springer Science+Business Media
233 Spring Street
New York, NY 10013
www.springer.com

Library of Congress Control Number:
2008938225

Manufactured in the United States of America.
Printed on acid-free paper.

ISBN 978-0-387-79475-4   e-ISBN 978-0-387-79476-1

"What mattered to me as person living with HIV was to be told that HIV did not cause AIDS. That was nice. Of course, it was like printing money when the economy is not doing well. Or pissing in your pants when the weather is too cold. Comforting for a while but disastrous in the long run."

–Winstone Zulu, Zambian AIDS
Activist and former denialist

Author Disclaimer of Potential Conspiracy Involvement

Seth C. Kalichman has never taken financial support from any pharmaceutical company, although he has accepted pens and key chains from Pfizer sales reps at conventions. He has also not applied for or received funding from the Bill and Melinda Gates foundation; however, this book was word processed in Microsoft Word. Kalichman is also a U2 fanatic and purchases Product (Red) whenever possible. When he is not working to understand AIDS denialism, Kalichman conducts HIV/AIDS prevention and treatment research in Atlanta and South Africa. His research is funded by the National Institutes of Heath but he has never met nor communicated with Robert Gallo. Kalichman is a Professor of Psychology at the University of Connecticut and is therefore an employee of The State. He is the editor of the journal *AIDS and Behavior,* published by Springer Science & Business Media.

The author is donating all of his royalties from sales of this book to the Family Treatment Fund administered by Massachusetts General Hospital to purchase antiretroviral medications for people living with HIV/AIDS in Africa. Visit the Family Treatment Fund website at http://www.shallwego.net/ftf/index.htm.

Foreword

HIV causes AIDS. This is not a controversial claim but an established fact, based on more than 25 years of science. Yet a small group of AIDS denialists claims that HIV is harmless, and that the antiretroviral drugs used to fight it cause, rather than treat, AIDS. They believe that the pharmaceutical industry has somehow conspired with thousands of doctors and scientists, to invent a disease as a means of selling harmful drugs. Such talk sounds to most of us like lunacy. But the sad fact is that AIDS denialism has emerged as a genuine menace to global public health including in the United States and, particularly, in South Africa.

AIDS denialism gained such currency with former President Thabo Mbeki of South Africa that his administration was, until recently, reluctant to expand access to antiretroviral drugs. This delay cost thousands of lives and to this day only a third of those needing antiretrovirals actually receive them. This response is poor by the standards of middle-income countries, but it is especially troublesome in South Africa, which has more HIV-positive people than any other country.

American AIDS denialists are partly to blame for South Africa's unfortunate history of AIDS policy. Peter Duesberg, the leading AIDS denialist, and his small band of supporters was invited by Thabo Mbeki to serve on his presidential panel on AIDS. These denialists rejected all the evidence presented to them about the efficacy of using antiretrovirals for the prevention of mother to child transmission. This resulted in policy deadlock and further delayed the use of antiretrovirals either for prevention or treatment. Even after the panel had completed its work, the Health Minister, Manto Tshabalala-Msimang, continued to support AIDS denialists (even engaging one of them as an advisor), to promote unproven alternative nutritional remedies and to denigrate antiretrovirals as poison. Several prominent South Africans died of AIDS after opting to change their diets instead of taking antiretrovirals.

The health minister also failed to take steps against another AIDS denialist, Matthias Rath, for running illegal clinical trials in African townships in which AIDS patients were asked to go off antiretrovirals and onto vitamins instead. It was only after a protracted legal battle fought by the Treatment Action Campaign that these trials were recently declared illegal. In the past, South Africa's Medicines Control Council acted swiftly to curb such abuses but the power of this body was steadily eroded by the Health Minister. AIDS denialism now underpins a lucrative nutritional supplements industry that had the tacit, and sometimes active, support of the Mbeki administration.

By courting the AIDS denialists, President Mbeki has increased their stature in the United States. He lent credibility to Christine Maggiore, a Californian who campaigns against using antiretrovirals to prevent mother to child transmission, when he was photographed meeting her. Two years later, Ms. Maggiore gave birth to a daughter who tragically died at age 3 of what the coroner concluded was an AIDS-related infection. Mother-to-child transmission is now rare in the United States, thanks to the widespread use of preventive therapy and the activities of organizations like the National Institutes of Health and the Elizabeth Glaser Pediatric AIDS Foundation. Sadly, this is not so in South Africa, where many children are born infected and then face short, painful lives.

Until recently, AIDS researchers and activists in the United States tended to regard the denialists with derision, assuming they would fade away. Unfortunately, this has not happened. Journalists like Celia Farber continue to promote the denialist view and keep them in the public eye. More disturbingly, she and Duesberg received awards during "whistleblower week" in Washington during 2008. This indicates that AIDS denialists have not only been capable of convincing vulnerable AIDS patients to go off their medications, but have also managed to win over certain public opinion makers with their misrepresentations and erroneous point of view. There is a real risk that a new generation of Americans could be persuaded that HIV either does not exist or is harmless, that safe sex is not important and that they do not need to protect their children from this deadly virus. A resurgence of denialism in the United States would have far reaching effects on the global AIDS pandemic, just as it already has in South Africa.

Who are these AIDS denialists and what motivates them to pursue their deadly campaign? Seth Kalichman tackles this difficult topic here in this very useful, timely and insightful book. He provides an engaging portrait of the key AIDS denialists in the United States, showing that they are, at heart, "suspicious thinkers" prone to conspiracy theories and other wacky beliefs. This exposé is very important because all too often innocent people are lead to believe that there is a genuine "scientific debate" over AIDS. There is not. We know more about HIV and how it causes AIDS than we know about any other pathogen. AIDS denialists promote the illusion of scientific debate. Seth Kalichman shatters that illusion by pointing to their erroneous forms of reasoning and unscientific approaches. Everyone should read this book.

Nicoli Nattrass
Cape Town, South Africa

Preface

My strange journey into HIV/AIDS denialism started with a seemingly random event. As the editor of the behavioral science research journal *AIDS and Behavior* I sent an email to everyone who had ever been asked to provide peer reviews for papers submitted to the journal requesting that they update their contact information. Psychologist Kelly Brennan-Jones at the State University of New York in Brockport replied to my email and said that she had no idea who I was, why I sent her the request, and asked me to remove her from the journal database. How she got my email was simply that I had asked her to review a paper some time back to which she had declined. As an expert in the study of relationships, I knew her work dating back to my years in graduate school. I knew Kelly Brennan-Jones was trained at a superlative university by some of the best social psychologists in the country. When I reminded her of the request to review for the journal and asked if she would consider reviewing in the future, she promptly directed me to an internet link telling me to read the information there if I was interested in knowing what she thought of AIDS. The link was to the David Crowe's Alberta Reappraising AIDS Society website which posted her August 2007 article "The HIV/AIDS Myth: A Review of [Peter] Duesberg's *Inventing the AIDS Virus*". My reaction was one of absolute outrage. I mean I was really angry. I was in an emotional upheaval. I surprised everyone around me, including myself, by my seemingly irrational reaction. How could someone I knew to be intelligent, well-trained as a scientist at a respectable university and in a position of influence over college students endorse a book that everyone surely knows is outdated, biased, and of little more value than that worthy of a doorstop?

Having dedicated my entire adult life to preventing the suffering caused by HIV/AIDS, I realize that HIV disease is very complex. People who test HIV positive as well as those who care for them will gladly grasp at the idea that HIV does not cause AIDS. Who wouldn't? Peter Duesberg, and all the denialists who have followed him, offers that very false hope. Repackaged by what has become a movement of denialism and propped up by a pseudoscientific enterprise, the idea that HIV does not cause AIDS has floated around for nearly 20 years. It just does not go away. In fact, the movement grows stronger in every country that is suffering a significant AIDS problem. For some, like many of us in the United States, it is easy to ignore HIV/AIDS denialism because its followers are invisible to us. For others, like my friends in South Africa, it is impossible to ignore. People living with HIV/AIDS in every country are vulnerable to the confusion and disinformation propagated by a small group of denialists whether by their books, brochures, or Internet postings. Reading that HIV does not cause AIDS can dissuade people from getting tested for HIV, lead HIV infected people to ignore their HIV positive test result, and persuade some to reject antiretroviral therapies in place of vitamins and nutritional supplements. These are not hypothetical situations. Real people are facing a life threatening disease that can be effectively treated. Realizing that all AIDS scientists should take action to counter the claims of HIV/AIDS denialism, I decided to write this book.

To understand HIV/AIDS denialism, I had to start from scratch. Like nearly every AIDS scientist, I have ignored denialism. I suppose you could say I was in denial about denialism. I knew it was out there, but I pushed it to the back of my mind. To begin my journey into the world of HIV/AIDS denialism I dived into books, magazines, and most of all, the Internet to learn all angles. Still, it seemed insufficient. Getting to know the denialists not just their papers seemed essential. So I started corresponding, conversing, and visiting the insiders of HIV/AIDS denialism. I posed questions and gained insight into the inner workings of denialism. Most of those I contacted responded to me. Not really knowing who I am, they took me under their wing to enlighten me about the truth about AIDS. I have been left with no doubt that the AIDS Rethinkers really truly believe that HIV does not cause AIDS. In their minds, the propagation of the HIV=AIDS myth is the product of a government conspiracy in cahoots with a multibillion dollar pharmaceutical scam. They actually believe that antiretroviral medications are toxic poison. In their minds, they have not been duped like everyone else into thinking that HIV causes AIDS and one day the AIDS orthodoxy will crumble on its own lies. I looked one denialist in her eyes and asked her if she really believes these things about AIDS and she said without any hesitation "yes I do". It is through these cordial and inquisitive exchanges that I learned most about this problem.

My relationships with denialists created some complicated arrangements that allowed me to experience denialism face-to-face. I often felt more like a journalist than a scientist, giving me a glimpse of how it must feel when denialist journalists delve into science. Still, it is important that I say that the denialists who interacted with me did not seem evil. They are deeply skeptical of science and untrusting of government and big business. Some are surely misguided and others seem to foolishly believe that they understand everything there was to know about AIDS. But I did not find them evil in the sense they were intent on harming people, even though their actions surely are. Of course, those I have come to see as malevolent – the vitamin pushers, con men, and angry academics are the ones who did not respond to may attempts to contact them.

I gained as much of an inside view of HIV/AIDS denialism as I could. Obviously, at times I have felt quite sympathetic to some of the denialists. I am not sure if these feelings reflected something of a Stockholm syndrome, where I was identifying with those who seemed to become my psychological captures. In retrospect, I think I was just struggling to understand them as best I could, an understanding I have tried to convey in this book.

Writing this book posed some rather unique challenges. I have tried to remain objective and balanced in my examination of what the denialists are saying and who they are. Difficult as it may be, I have tried to take these guys seriously; even if not what they are saying then why they are saying it. I have also tried to avoid ad homonym attacks by focusing more on what the denialists are saying than who they are. But that too was difficult. This book is a psychological perspective on denialism, so the denialists themselves are central to the story. In this case, the messengers may be as important as the messages. I also struggled with what to consider science vs. pseudoscience. Including someone and their work under the rubric of pseudoscience was never taken lightly. As a guide, I used standard definitions of pseudoscience and I spoke with colleagues and collaborators of those in question. I know that no one included in the discussion of pseudoscience, and denialist journalism for that matter, will appreciate these labels. Nevertheless, I believe that the categorization is valid and meaningful. In a related matter, I spend considerable time discussing peer review, for all its value and deficiencies. When considering work as scientific and pseudoscientific, I considered whether articles had been peer reviewed. For this, I also relied on co-authors as well as the authors themselves to tell me if their work had been peer reviewed. Although some of the articles I discuss as pseudoscience did appear in peer reviewed journals, it is my understanding that the specific articles did not undergo peer review.

Another element of this book that I particularly grappled with was managing its citations and sources. I found myself wanting to cite numerous studies that support the facts that HIV causes AIDS and that antiretrovirals extend lives and prevent babies from becoming infected to debunk denialist claims. In doing so, I would have lost my footing and the very point of this book. This is not a book about AIDS and how it is caused by HIV. Rather, this is a book about HIV/AIDS denialism. I did not write this book to answer the denialist claims, but rather to offer insight into their wacky and destructive world. I have maintained an electronic library of all my sources that I used to write this book should any of the websites be terminated. Given the nature of the topic, a lot of my sources are from Internet websites. Knowing that websites come and go, especially those on the fringe, I printed all of my sources as portable documents. I am happy to share these sources. In the chapter notes, I do not always indicate dates of websites accessed because I verified downloaded websites on a single day, February 13, 2008, unless otherwise noted. To request my sources and to learn more about my experiences infiltrating the world of AIDS denialism visit the Denying AIDS blog at http://denyingaids.blogspot.com/

Personally, I have come to view this book as just one straw on the back of HIV/AIDS denialism. A back that will not break until the public is educated to differentiate science from pseudoscience, facts from fraud. Denialism is defeated when credible science is effectively communicated to a trusting and critically minded public. My goal has been to offer a psychological perspective on what is essentially a psychological and social phenomenon. I do not view myself as an anti-denialist waging war against denialism. To the contrary, I am trying to understand what the denialists are saying and why anyone would believe them. As my South African friend Nicoli Nattrass suggested, in writing this book I am offering a psychological autopsy of HIV/AIDS denialism. Although I find the problem of HIV/AIDS denialism fascinating, it is not my aspiration to immerse myself in the world of denialism any longer. I will now return to the less glamorous and mundane world of AIDS prevention and treatment research, where there are far fewer dramas and conspiracies to contend with.

Odd as it is, I find myself drawing this project to a close sitting and writing these words on the steps of Peter Duesberg's laboratory at the Donner Building in the shade of the beautiful trees on the lovely UC Berkeley campus. I suppose stranger things have happened, just not to me.

S.C. Kalichman
Storrs, CT

Acknowledgments

I am indebted to Bill Tucker at Springer for his endless support of this project. Bill is a wonderful editor and a terrific human being whose commitment to publishing sound AIDS science has surely saved lives. I also owe enormous thanks to Paul Farrell for his critical reading and editorial direction. Without Paul, this would have been a different and far less interesting project. I also want to thank my long time mentor Jeff Kelly for finding the idea for this book interesting and encouraging me to pursue it. Thanks to David Bangsberg at Harvard University for being my go-to-guy on matters of HIV and AIDS that were beyond my reach. Also thanks to Leickness Simbayi for opening my world to South Africa and to Yolande Shean for couriering Mark Gevisser's biography of Thabo Mbeki for me across the Atlantic. Others who encouraged me to delve into the world of HIV/AIDS denialism despite their concerns for my mental health and career, are Moira Kalichman my partner and comrade and Lisa Eaton the greatest graduate student anyone could work with. Thanks to Demetria Cain, Chauncey Cherry and the entire Southeast HIV/AIDS Research and Evaluation Project team for tolerating my ranting about mythical monsters, government conspiracies, and alien scientists. I am forever indebted to my writing buddy Hannah Kalichman, who has taken great interest in the strange and unusual that is so much a part of this project.

In writing this book, I have also gained enormous support from a group of anti-denialists. I cannot thank them enough for opening their minds and pointing me toward invaluable resources. Nicoli Nattrass at the University of Cape Town wrote the first book on HIV/AIDS denialism that inspired me to write this book and provided critical feedback on an early draft. Nicoli set a very high standard to follow and this book should be seen as an adjunct to hers. I am also grateful to Nicoli for writing the Foreword and providing a South African perspective. Thanks to John Moore of Cornell University for his insights into denialism and to Nathan Geffen of the Treatment Action Campaign for encouraging this project and pointing me toward Michael

Shermer and all those weird things that people believe. Other members of aidstruth.org, especially Nick Bennett, Brian Foley, and Bob Funkhouser were very generous in giving me their time and answering my questions. I also appreciate Mike Merson, Mark Wainberg, Jon Cohen and Martin Delaney for the time they took from their busy schedules to correspond with me about their views and experiences. I am grateful to Salim Abdool Karim, Glenda Gray and James McIntyre for sharing their experiences on the 2000 South African Presidential AIDS Panel and providing me with some valuable historically important documents. I am also indebted to the world's greatest political cartoonist, South Africa's Jonathan Shapiro (Zapiro), for giving me permission to include his art in this book. I also thank the Starbucks in Storrs, the De Luca Café in Cape Town, and Berkeley Espresso for giving me the space to work. I am also indebted to Joey for taking me places I could not have otherwise gone. Finally, I want to thank the HIV/AIDS denialist mentors with whom I had numerous email exchanges and conversations. I will leave them unnamed to protect identities, but I cannot thank them enough for their willingness to take me in even without knowing who I am.

This book is dedicated to the memory of Dan Dunable, longtime Atlanta AIDS activist, HIV treatment educator, and compassionate advocate against AIDS denialism.

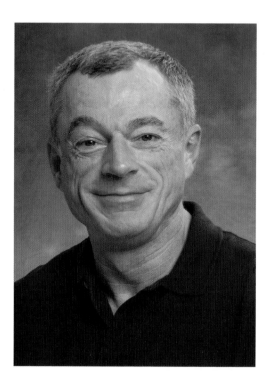

Note on Terminology

Throughout this book I refer to denialism with specific reference to HIV/ AIDS denialism. However, repeated use of HIV/AIDS denialism made for a cumbersome read. I therefore use the term "denialism" to exclusively refer to HIV/AIDS denialism. When referring to other forms of denialism I clearly indicate doing so, such as Holocaust denialism or 9/11 denialism.

Contents

HIV/AIDS Denialism Is Alive and Well

Every epidemic throughout history has had its "denialists." Some epidemics have been blamed on rats, some on foreigners, Jews, or other disfavored local ethnic groups. Very often, epidemics have been blamed on the people who suffered from them, their illness being seen as some kind of moral failure. Sound familiar?
Martin Delaney, AIDS Activist, 2000

"Are they still around?" That is what nearly everyone in the United States said, when I told them about this book. They found it difficult to believe that after all these years, anyone still questions the cause of AIDS. Scientists have admittedly found it easy to ignore denialism. We typically dismiss HIV/AIDS denialists as a small group of rogue journalists and unstable troublemakers. Sadly, people who work on HIV/AIDS often fail to realize that denialism is a significant problem because denialists dissuade those affected by AIDS from seeking help. People who are lured to denialism are invisible to AIDS service and treatment providers. Denialism – like stigma, sexism, and homophobia – undermines the fight against AIDS. At the very least, denialism diverts attention and resources from the global AIDS disaster. At its worst, it disinforms affected populations about the importance of prevention, the necessity of HIV testing, and the availability of life-prolonging treatments. At its core, denialism is destructive because it undermines trust in science, medicine, and public health.

In this Chapter, I define HIV/AIDS denialism, focusing on what it is and what it is not. At the start, it is essential to distinguish between denialism and the psychological process of denial, the doubt that patients often express about their medical care, and the important role of dissidence in science. Let us begin by looking at psychological denial, doubt and the difficult patient, and dissidence.

Denial

In its truest sense, denial is a passive coping response. In psychological terms, denial is an emotional defense mechanism. A nearly universal immediate reaction to trauma, denial involves a subconscious refusal to believe the unbelievable. Denial occurs when we confront something too painful or frightening to face, providing a protective buffer zone, a time and space to assimilate a stressor or trauma into one's sense of reality. Perhaps the best-known account of psychological denial is Elizabeth Kubler-Ross' classic description of how people cope with a terminal illness. In her five stages of coping with death and dying, Kubler-Ross places denial as the first, necessary stage of coping with mortality, exemplified by the reaction, "No, not me." This stage of denial is the time when people want medical tests re-run, when they refuse to return to their doctor, or when they seek to escape reality through alcohol or drugs. The National Cancer Institute describes denial in this way:

> When you were first diagnosed, you may have had trouble believing or accepting the fact that you have cancer. This is called denial. Denial can be helpful because it can give you time to adjust to your diagnosis. Denial can also give you time to feel hopeful and better about the future.[1]

Stanley Cohen, in his classic book on denial, describes the fundamental paradox of simultaneously knowing and not knowing. People must have some awareness of the threat they are denying, or there could be no denial response. Yet denial keeps us from consciously knowing.

Denial is a normal and perhaps universal psychological response to trauma. As a coping mechanism, denial shields our emotions from a harsh reality. People diagnosed with HIV/AIDS, who are experiencing denial, are in the process of coping with the traumatic experience of testing positive for HIV. The same can be true for those close to someone who tests HIV positive – a friend or lover, a parent, a sibling, or a child. Interestingly, those who are in psychological denial are the very people to whom denialists pose the greatest threat. Denial is perhaps best understood as passive avoidance. Though denial can, for a time, serve very well as a way of adjusting to the truth, to making one's peace, it can, when it goes on too long, become maladaptive, keeping us from moving on to active coping strategies.

We should expect anyone who confronts a serious medical diagnosis, such as a positive indication of HIV infection, to respond with denial. Denial should not, however, become a fixed state; rather, it should be a fluid, dynamic process that changes with time. When denial extends for longer than a few months, people are more likely to delay or completely avoid opportunities for medical treatment. The National Cancer Institute states, "Sometimes, denial is a serious problem. If it lasts too long, it can keep you from getting the treatment you need. It can also be a problem when other people deny that you have cancer, even after you have accepted it."[2] In fact, maladaptive denial is a form of mental illness. Psychiatrists define maladaptive denial as:

> The persistence of a maladaptive mode of experiencing, perceiving, evaluating, and responding to one's own health status, despite the fact that a doctor has provided a lucid and accurate appraisal of the situation and management to be followed...[3]

The most extreme case of maladaptive denial is malignant denial, during which people completely ignore their physical condition, with potentially irreversible damage. There are clinical cases in medicine of women who have denied that they are pregnant up until the time they deliver their baby. Denial is a common feature of conditions that are unacceptable to one's self-identity, such as alcoholism, drug abuse, excessive gambling, sexual addictions, and eating disorders. With respect to HIV/AIDS, malignant denial occurs when a person tests HIV positive and continues to expose others to the virus through unprotected sex or sharing injection drug equipment. Avoiding doctors and refusing treatment are also hallmarks of malignant denial.

Malignant denial extends beyond a psychological safety net to ultimately threaten one's health. When malignant, the avoidance of denial permeates into health care and health decisions. Denialist propaganda and the false promises of quackery target those people who are most vulnerable, particularly those whose denial has become entrenched. People in denial are saying "this cannot be happening to me" and denialism responds with a resounding "you are right, it is not happening to you." Denialism feeds on those who are experiencing the very real and humanly understandable state of psychological denial.

An illustrative example of malignant denial in HIV/AIDS may be helpful. Perhaps the most public – even notorious – case involved a woman named Christine Maggiore. After testing HIV positive, she became involved in AIDS activism in Los Angeles. However, she later came to question whether HIV causes AIDS, influenced by the writings of rogue scientist Peter Duesberg and his associates. Christine Maggiore turned her AIDS activism toward denial and, in the course of time, toward what I am calling denialism. Maggiore wrote a book and her husband produced a movie that questions HIV as the cause of AIDS based on her experiences, started an organization around denialism, and has worked to discourage people from getting tested for HIV.

Maggiore has become the most visible and seemingly one of the most influential denialists in the United States. Her influence clearly must be in part due to the undeniably tragic circumstances of her life. However, it was her own denial that led to the tragedy: She avoided taking preventive action against transmitting HIV to her baby, Eliza Jane Scovill. The girl died of complications from AIDS at age 3. Maggiore's denial had become literally malignant. And then, in the months following her daughter's death, her stance morphed further into denialism: She set herself to actively misrepresenting and distorting and undermining AIDS science, medical programs, and public health policies. Refuting the report of the Los Angeles medical examiner, Maggiore was assisted by Mohammed Al-Bayati, an AIDS denialist and veterinary toxicologist, who said Eliza Jane actually died of an allergic reaction to the antibiotic *Amoxicillin*. The historical record shows that Christine Maggiore's denial caused harm first to herself, then to her daughter, and ultimately to who knows how many others, clearly illustrating the destructive progression from ordinary psychological denial to malignant denial to denialism.

Doubt and the Difficult Patient

Just as psychological denial can morph from a reasonable human-coping strategy to something much more dangerous and even sinister, so can doubt and the desire to be an involved and active patient turn from healthy, emotionally understandable, and even helpful impulses to something much less desirable and productive. When people come out of denial and accept their condition, it remains common to question medical decisions and even to doubt one's prognosis. Denial may even recur, to help patients retain hope. So again, we are faced with good motives, or at least emotionally comprehensible motives, providing a possible pathway to denialism.

Patients who ask questions and express doubt in their doctor's recommendations are the same patients who are most engaged in their care and actively participate in medical decisions. Research has shown that patients who actively engage in their care and probe their providers with challenging questions actually survive longer than those who are passive. But self-determined patients might also be difficult to manage, at least by some doctors, and may be particularly vulnerable to false claims and misinformation when exposed to denialists.

In addition to denial, people diagnosed with a serious illness may doubt the value of modern treatments. Doubt can lead to the refusal of treatment even when a person is not in denial. For example, many people with HIV infection believe it is better to wait before starting treatment, keeping as many of their options open for as long as possible. The strategy of delaying treatment paid off for many people who did not follow the recommendation to "hit HIV hard and early," back when doctors thought early treatment was the best plan. New treatments and treatment guidelines for HIV infection become available with unprecedented speed. In talking with people who have HIV/AIDS and have opted out of taking antiretroviral therapy, I have found some do so because they prefer holistic and natural remedies. In some cases, doctors reject natural remedies, as explained to me by one person who had been living with untreated HIV for over a decade:

> After years of thinking I should get tested for HIV I finally did. I made the decision after a former sex partner died of AIDS. I tested positive and soon after developed a couple of serious infections. Being a naturalist in terms of my health care my entire life, I chose to use herbal remedies to treat myself. But when I became quite ill I went to an AIDS specialist. My natural therapies weren't clearing up the problem, so I wanted to see if a doctor had any solutions. This doctor was totally out of touch with holistic health and healing and was not even open to the idea. The experience confirmed to me that I was on the right track.[4]

When I talk with people who have removed themselves from HIV treatment, they have said that their doctors resent their asking challenging questions. Whether accurate or not, the perception of a closed-minded physician is a likely reason for patients to opt out of care. However, these people, whom I categorize as difficult patients, are usually not in denial about their illness. They clearly recognize their condition and understand their treatment alternatives, but choose something different from the recommendations of their doctors. The difficult patient may, in a few instances, also be doubtful about his or her condition or its severity, but the main focus of their doubt tends to be on the recommended treatments.

Psychological denial, doubt, and the difficult patient do not fall under the general heading of what we will call denialism. However, patients who are in denial, those who doubt their doctor's recommendations, and those who are otherwise dissatisfied with and in some cases resist or decline medical care are the most vulnerable to the false claims of denialists.

Dissidence in Science

Consensus does not determine the truth, certainly not in science. Science does, however, move through a social process of truth-seeking in which facts are agreed upon. Any single observation or single experiment cannot determine facts in science. To trust an observation, an independent observer must repeat experiments done earlier and arrive at substantially the same results. When many independent observers record the same experimental results with their methods tightly controlled and under strict scrutiny, scientists may consider the observation true. In science, theories lead to questions, just the same as in philosophy. However, it is the accumulation of objective observations that differentiates science from philosophy. Scientific consensus occurs when independent scientists agree on the body of accumulated facts.

Scientists who hold views outside of the mainstream play an important role in truth seeking. Dissident scientists do not agree with the prevailing theory or do not accept the body of accumulated observations as fact. The importance of dissidence in science is unquestionable, with many celebrated examples throughout history. Revolutions in how we think about our world come from those who move science in new directions. We remember the dissident scientists who changed the way we think. Galileo Galilei changed how we view our universe. Albert Einstein changed how we contemplate space and time. Alfred Wegener changed how we think about the formation of our planet. Charles Darwin changed our view of life. Sigmund Freud changed how we view ourselves. Dissident scientists turn into revolutionaries when their thinking causes science to shift course. Science surely values diverse thinkers, dissent, disagreement, and vigorous debate. How those of us outside of a respective field of science distinguish between genuine dissidence and destructive attempts to undermine the science is a far more complicated matter.

The science of AIDS began in the early 1980s, when there were numerous theories proposed to account for this new disease – most centering on the lifestyle characteristics of the people first diagnosed. After all, the first AIDS cases were among gay men and people who used injection drugs. All of the first AIDS patients had become ill with rare illnesses. The strange clusters of diseases these patients suffered from resulted, scientists soon realized, from a collapsing immune system. Because of the ages and social characteristics of these first patients, it was readily apparent that the cause had to be an environmental agent rather than an inherited gene. It was common for men and women diagnosed with AIDS to have a history of drug abuse, even if they did not inject drugs. One early theory of AIDS stated that drugs were causing the immune system to fail. But soon hemophiliacs, including young children like Ryan White, who would become the icon for the indiscriminant affliction of HIV infection, were found to have the disease in statistically large numbers, so it became obvious that AIDS could not be the result of drug abuse. In addition, blood-transfusion recipients, like tennis star Arthur Ashe, were diagnosed. The medical reasons for the blood transfusions differed too much to consider any one of them the cause of AIDS. In 1984, the virus that causes AIDS was identified and ultimately named Human Immunodeficiency Virus. The only thing that links all of the gay men, drug users, commercial sex workers, hemophiliacs, blood-transfusion recipients, and others who have had AIDS whether they are in Los Angeles, New York, Paris, or Kampala Uganda is that they test positive for HIV infection.

Still, not all scientists agreed that the newly identified virus was the sole cause of AIDS. At the time, doctors knew little about HIV and how it destroys critical immune system cells. Peter Duesberg, a cancer researcher who had mapped the genetic makeup of a virus that is similar to HIV, disputed the predominant theory that a virus was causing AIDS. Duesberg, a respected – some would even say renowned – scientist at the University of California at Berkeley, believed that a single virus could not disable the immune system and cause AIDS. Departing sharply from the overwhelmingly prevalent scientific view, Duesberg said he believed that AIDS must result from drug abuse and other lifestyle factors. And he was not alone in proposing other causes. For example, Robert Root-Bernstein, a well-known and respected professor of life sciences at Michigan State University, proposed that HIV alone was not causing AIDS and that multiple factors must be at play to cause the collapse of the immune system. Well regarded and respected New York physician Joseph Sonnabend was among the first to care for the earliest cases of AIDS among gay men in New York City. He joined with Michael Callen to start the People with AIDS Health Group, one of the first HIV treatment advocacy organizations. Early on, Sonnabend stated that AIDS must have many causes, not a single source. Like nearly all other AIDS dissident scientists, Root-Bernstein and Sonnabend altered their views as the facts of AIDS became clear. In a 2006 statement on his changing views about AIDS, Root-Bernstein said the following:

> Both the camps that say HIV is a pussycat and the people who claim AIDS is all HIV are wrong....[but] the denialists make claims that are clearly inconsistent with existing studies. When I check the existing studies, I don't agree with their inter-pretation of the data, or, worse, I can't find the studies [at all].[5]

Similarly, Sonnabend clarified his views on AIDS over the years, stating in 2007:

> Some individuals who believe that HIV plays no role at all in AIDS have implied that I support their misguided views on AIDS causation by including inappropriate refer-ences to me in their literature and on their web sites. Before HIV was discovered and its association with AIDS established, I held the entirely appropriate view that the cause of AIDS was then unknown. I have successfully treated hundreds of AIDS patients with antiretroviral medications, and have no doubt that HIV plays a necessary role in this disease, a view that I have expressed publicly on several occasions. It is my view that the relationship of HIV to AIDS is of the same nature as that of almost all viruses to the diseases with which they are associated. It is thus similar to the relationship of the Hepatitis A, B and C viruses to clinical hepatitis, or poliovirus to poliomyelitis or the influenza viruses to influenza. In the same way HIV disease, including AIDS, is related to HIV as necessary for disease causation.[6]

Thus, as science moved forward into the 1990s and scientists discovered how HIV causes AIDS, most dissident views faded. Nearly all dissident scientists critically examined the evidence, adapted their views to accommodate the facts and moved on. Science is after all a forward-moving and evolving enterprise.

But some dissidents did not waver in the face of mounting evidence. They seemed more invested in holding on to the rightness of their initial views than they were in following the evidence, wherever it may have led. In doing so, they turned the corner from dissidence to denialism.

What Is HIV/AIDS Denialism?

Denialism actively propagates myths, misconceptions, and misinformation to distort and refute reality. A formal definition of denialism that I find particularly fitting comes from a group that tracks denialist activity on the Internet. They define denialism as follows:

> The employment of rhetorical tactics to give the appearance of argument or legitimate debate, when in actuality there is none. These false arguments are used when one has few or no facts to support one's viewpoint against a scientific consensus or against overwhelming evidence to the contrary. They are effective in distracting from actual useful debate using emotionally appealing, but ultimately empty and illogical assertions. Examples of common topics in which Denialists employ their tactics include: Creationism/Intelligent Design, Global Warming Denialism, Holocaust Denial, HIV/AIDS Denialism, 9/11 conspiracies, tobacco carcinogenecity denialism (the first organized corporate campaign), anti-vaccina-tion/mercury autism denialism and anti-animal testing/animal rights extremist denialism. Denialism spans the ideological spectrum, and is about tactics rather than politics or partisanship.[7]

Denialism is the outright rejection of science and medicine. It involves actively contradicting and disregarding medical advice. It is steady state. Denialism is not open to criticism, and it evades modification. Denialism is only open to additional evidence supporting its tenets, and such evidence most often comes from the misuse of science and from pseudoscience. AIDS denialists, often for the sake of personal preservation or recognition, hold fast to old ideas in the face of new evidence.

One of the main features of denialism is a tendency to defend one's position at all costs, rather than to openly consider others' points of view. Proving oneself right seems to take precedence over following the evidence, even when that evidence seems to contradict one's own position and lead closer to the truth. Denialists refute new facts and remain stuck in the past.

A feature of denialism, at least at its root, is the tendency to think of the denialist position as beleaguered, and under attack and in a minority that has to stave off the assaults of the vast wrong-thinking majority. As a consequence, those involved in denialism often, in the other justifications for their position, declare their strong allegiance to the principle of free speech. Interestingly, then, denialists often set themselves up as plucky underdogs, battling for their right to speak the truth against a tide of misinformation and, as often as not, conspiracies aimed at keeping them silent.

The kind of distorted thinking inherent in denialism can be brought into clearer focus when it is compared to other types of denialism. It is important to note that denialism is a label that no one appreciates receiving. I recognize that it is an emotionally charged term, as expressed by denialist blogger Liam Scheff:

> Denialism is a term, carefully chosen for meaning and emotional response. The term asks the reader to equate those, like myself, who look at "HIV tests" and read that they are neither specific, standardized, or able to diagnose any particular infection, and who therefore question their ethical utility – and those who deny the German/Jewish Holocaust of the 1930s and 1940s. It is not a mistake that the term is used. It is used specifically, to cause anyone with any sensitivity to run screaming from the argument, lest they make the terrible mistake of perhaps falling into "denialism."[8]

Scheff is certainly right that the link to Holocaust denialism means that the word is emotionally charged. Still, I defend my use of the term because I believe it best describes the rejection of objective reality to sustain a flawed, hurtful, and ultimately dangerous belief system. As Scheff points out, deniers and denialists are both terms that describe people who refuse to accept the historical reality of Nazi Germany and the Holocaust. There are also 9/11 denialists and those who deny that man ever walked on the moon. Denialism emerges from defiance against objective historical records or, in the case of AIDS, defiance against established science. Still, those who doubt that the Holocaust or 9/11 ever happened do not identify themselves as "denialists" but rather "truth seekers." The journalist Celia Farber, who has chronicled much of Peter Duesberg's thinking on AIDS, expresses her outrage at those who call her a denialist:

> Attempts to rigorously test the ruling medical hypothesis of the age are met not with reasoned debate but with the rhetoric of moral blackmail: Peter Duesberg has the blood of African AIDS babies on his hands. Duesberg is evil, a scientific psychopath. He should be imprisoned. Those who wish to engage the AIDS research establishment in the sort of causality debate that is carried on in most other branches of scientific endeavor are tarred as AIDS "denialists," as if skepticism about the pathogenicity of a retrovirus were the moral equivalent of denying that the Nazis slaughtered 6 million Jews.[9]

It is plain to see, however, that HIV/AIDS denialists represent just one variant of the broader phenomenon of denialism, sharing common characteristics with Holocaust Deniers, 9/11 Truthers, and others who refuse to accept an indisputable historical record. At the core of denialism is mistrust – in the case of HIV/AIDS, the mistrust is of science and medicine. Scholars have identified the characteristics of political extremists and fringe groups that promote Holocaust denialism. These same characteristics apply equally well to HIV/AIDS denialism. First, extremist groups hold an absolute certainty that they are the sole bearers of "The Truth." For HIV/AIDS denialists, the truth is that HIV is a harmless virus that cannot possibly cause disease, and that anti-HIV medications amount to nothing more than poison, DNA terminators that can themselves cause AIDS. Second, extremist groups believe that governments are under the control of conspiring forces. In the case of HIV/AIDS denialism, the power of Big Pharma and the medical establishment have corrupted the National Institutes of Health and biomedical sciences in general. A third characteristic of extremists is a hatred for its opponents, often seen as conspiring with their enemies. HIV/AIDS denialists attack the most visible scientists; especially those who are widely exposed in the media as well as those who have publicly debunked their rhetoric. Fourth, extremists deny basic civil liberties to those whose views they see as their enemies. Ironically, denialists censor science by cherry-picking results of research while claiming to be the victims of censorship themselves, and often claiming that their rights to free expression are being systematically thwarted. Finally, denialists, as do extremists, indulge in irresponsible accusations and character assassination. As expected, denialists refer to AIDS scientists and medical specialists as Nazis, the mafia, and murderers.

A paranoid flare that characterizes conspiracy theorists is also apparent among denialists. Suspicious thinking permeates much of denialism. AIDS scientists typically avoid denialists and marginalizing them has likely helped to fuel their paranoia. Actual experiences have reinforced denialists' beliefs that the establishment is conspiring against them. I am sure that some of my own actions in researching this book will be touted as evidence that the AIDS orthodoxy is out to get them. One denialist, on account of his experience at an AIDS conference, offers a typical example:

> Early on it was clear that certain people at the meeting already knew of me. They avoided me. Others, though, initially showed interest when I raised my objections. It was obvious that these problems were not new to them, they had just never discussed them before – or been around anyone who wanted to. However, once these potential allies continued the discussions with people like Markowitz – scientists with status and influence – then they as well avoided me from then on. I found it a lonely business, acting like a scientist at an AIDS conference.[10]

Psychologist Michael Shermer is the leading authority on Holocaust denialism, and he has found that Holocaust deniers' "fallacies of reasoning are eerily similar to those of other fringe groups, such as creationists."[11] Remarkably, these same personality features that Shermer describe in Holocaust deniers are immediately recognizable among HIV/AIDS denialists. First, denialism concentrates on opponents' weak points without making definitive statements about their own position. In HIV/AIDS denialism, without a shred of credible evidence to the contrary, there is an incessant call for the one study that proves that HIV causes AIDS while not recognizing the thousands of studies that accumulate to irrefutably show that HIV causes AIDS. Even knowing the complexity of HIV and the barriers it poses to vaccines, Peter Duesberg looked me dead in the eyes and said that failure to achieve an HIV vaccine means that an infectious agent cannot be the cause of AIDS. Second, denialists exploit errors made by AIDS scientists, implying that a few errors detected in a mass of work calls into question the entire scientific enterprise. One example I discuss at length in Chapter 3 is a reference citation error in a figure showing the course of HIV disease, posted at the National Institutes of Health AIDS web site. David Crowe, a Canadian journalist, identified the error and used it as the basis for tracing the history of the graph, claiming that the process of HIV-causing AIDS shown in the graph is false. Crowe exploits what amounts to a clerical error to support a conspiracy theory that implicates leading AIDS scientist Anthony Fauci and the National Institutes of Health. Denialists also commonly use quotations taken out of context from prominent mainstream sources to bolster their own position. This strategy is ubiquitous in denialism and includes morphing science into pseudoscience, cherry-picking, and relying on a single study – the so-called single-study fallacy. Denialists warp the findings of a single study to support their views and exploit discrepancies with past research. The fourth flaw in reasoning common among denialists is mistaking genuine honest debate in a given field as a dispute about the existence of the very field itself. Finally, denialists focus on the unknown and ignore the known. They emphasize research findings that fit their views and discount those that do not. For example, in HIV/AIDS, denialists concentrate on side effects of HIV treatments while ignoring the declining hospitalizations and increasing longevity among those who receive treatment.

Holocaust and HIV/AIDS denialism share other common features. For both, millions of people died with the vast majority of Holocaust historians and AIDS scientists confirming the causes. The enormity of human suffering caused by the Holocaust and that of a plague, like AIDS, offers a platform for denialism. Another commonality is that conspiracy theories drive both Holocaust and HIV/AIDS denialism. There are striking similarities in rhetoric, using selected excerpts from credible documents and calling for a debate on matters for which there is universal agreement. Denialist groups of all types claim mounting controversy and the need for a debate. Both Holocaust and HIV/AIDS denialism have established their own publication outlets, such as the *Journal for Historical Review* for Holocaust denialism and *Continuum* magazine in HIV/AIDS denialism. There are full-length films produced by both movements, *The Truth Behind the Gates of Auschwitz*, produced by David Cole for Holocaust denialism and *HIV=AIDS: Fact or Fraud*, produced by Gary Null and *The Other Side of AIDS* produced by Eric Paulson and Robert Leppo for HIV/AIDS denialism. The major deniers of the Holocaust are knowledgeable of World War II history and are on the fringes of academia, just as the major HIV/AIDS denialists are well versed in the science of AIDS. Denialists of all types seize opportunities by political leaders who express support for their denialism, as has occurred in 2006 by Iran's President Mahmoud Ahmadinejad expressing doubt that the Holocaust occurred and President Thabo Mbeki of South Africa expressing doubt that HIV causes AIDS.

Those we call denialists generally prefer to be called dissidents. Perhaps, behind this preference are the crusading religious and political overtones associated with dissidence. Heretic is another term that may better capture the intent. But still, I preferred the term denialist rather than "denier" because it better represents the psychological process of malignant denial that is inherent in some denialism. Most denialists acknowledge the global AIDS problem but dispute that it is caused by HIV. I therefore use the term "HIV/AIDS denialism" to recognize that most current denialists refute HIV as the cause of AIDS while not necessarily disputing the existence of AIDS itself. A prominent group of denialists referred to as the Perth Group even bolster my rationale by stating the following:

> Let us make it clear that we are not AIDS denialists. That is, we do not deny that in 1981 a syndrome involving a high frequency of KS [Kaposi's sarcoma] and a number of opportunistic infections was identified in gay men and subsequently became known as AIDS. What we are doing and have been doing from the very beginning is to question the accepted cause of AIDS and to put forward an alternative theory for the cause of AIDS.[12]

HIV/AIDS denialism is therefore what Stanley Cohen refers to as interpretive denial. Most denialists do not dispute the objective fact of AIDS. Rather they believe an alternative view of reality. In interpretive denial, the raw facts of events are accepted but given a different meaning from what seems apparent to others. Cohen offers examples where the denier may say, "this was population exchange, not ethnic cleansing" or "the arms deal was not illegal, and it was not really even an arms deal."[13] In the case of HIV/AIDS denialism, the denialists say "AIDS is not caused by a single virus, there may not even be such a virus." Cohen states that word exchanges serve to reclassify events or objects, such as calling HIV treatments, "toxic poisons," or saying the causes of AIDS are "drugs and poverty."

I did however consider delusion as an alternative term for denialism. The psychiatric definition of a delusion is a false belief based on incorrect inference about external reality that is firmly sustained despite what almost everybody else believes and despite what constitutes incontrovertible and obvious evidence to the contrary. The belief is not one ordinarily accepted by other members of the person's culture or subculture (e.g., it is not an article of religious faith). I considered using the term delusion because the belief that HIV does not cause AIDS is easily refutable by a body of scientific evidence that spans thousands of research findings accepted as fact by thousands of scientists. Yet the belief that HIV does not cause AIDS persists in the face of the evidence, certainly bringing to mind delusional thinking. However, beliefs that HIV does not cause AIDS do not always occur within the context of a psychiatric condition, so the use of the term delusion is not appropriate. Believing that HIV does not cause AIDS can have many motives, none of which may be indicative of a mental illness. HIV/AIDS denialism therefore seems the most accurate descriptive term for refuting that HIV causes AIDS.

In summary, denialism is to denial as activism is to action. Like the activist, the denialist seeks to spread "The Truth" about AIDS. But denialists then cross over from merely informing others of alternative views on AIDS to actively campaigning to persuade people. Chapters 3 and 4 focus on the pseudoscientific basis of denialism and the promotional and persuasive strategies of denialists.

Suspicious Minds

At its very core, denialism is deeply embedded in a sense of mistrust. Most obviously, we see suspicion in denialist conspiracy theories (see Chapter 4). Most conspiracy theories grow out of suspicions about corruptions in government, industry, science, and medicine, all working together in some grand sinister plot. Psychologically, suspicion is the central feature of paranoid personality, and it is not overreaching to say that some denialists demonstrate this extreme. Suspicious thinking can be understood as a filter through which the world is interpreted, where attention is driven toward those ideas and isolated anecdotes that confirm one's preconceived notions of wrong doing. Suspicious thinkers are predisposed to see themselves as special or to hold some special knowledge.

Psychotherapist David Shapiro in his classic book *Neurotic Styles* describes the suspicious thinker. Just as we see in denialism, suspiciousness is not easily penetrated by facts or evidence that counter individuals' pre-conceived worldview. Just as Shapiro describes in the suspicious personality, the denialist selectively attends to information that bolsters his or her own beliefs. Denialists exhibit suspicious thinking when they manipulate objective reality to fit within their beliefs. It is true that all people are prone to fit the world into their sense of reality, but the suspicious person distorts reality and does so with an uncommon rigidity. The parallel between the suspicious personality style and denialism is really quite compelling. As described by Shapiro,

> A suspicious person is a person who has something on his mind. He looks at the world with fixed and preoccupying expectation, and he searches repetitively, and only, for confirmation of it. He will not be persuaded to abandon his suspicion of some plan of action based on it. On the contrary, he will pay no attention to rational arguments except to find in them some aspect or feature that actually confirms his original view. Anyone who tries to influence or persuade a suspicious person will not only fail, but also, unless he is sensible enough to abandon his efforts early will, himself, become an object of the original suspicious idea.[14]

The rhetoric of denialism clearly reveals a deeply suspicious character. In denialism, the science of AIDS is deconstructed to examine evidence taken out of context by non-scientists. The evidence is assimilated into one's beliefs that HIV does not cause AIDS, that HIV tests are invalid, that the science is corrupt, and aimed to profit Big Pharma.

Various denialist rhetorical techniques speak to suspiciousness, such as morphing science into pseudoscience, using overly technological terminology, and cherry picked research findings. All of these devices are employed in the service of self-perpetuating beliefs. As noted by Shapiro, the suspicious person "does not pay attention to the apparent facts, but, instead he or she pays sharp attention to any aspect of them or their presentation that lends confirmation to his original suspicious idea." The suspicious person constructs a subjective world based on "significant" clues with a complete loss of appreciation for the context. Shapiro also discusses the suspicious person as having encapsulated delusions, limited in content and type. Encapsulated delusions fit what we see in denialism, where a person can be grounded in reality in nearly every facet of his or her life and yet have a circumscribed entrenched belief system that is not reflective of reality and not refutable by facts.

The insights offered by Shapiro are that denialists are not "lying" in the way that most anti-denialists portray them. The cognitive style of the denialist represents a warped sense of reality for sure, explaining why arguing or debating with a denialist gets you no where. But the denialist is not the evil plotter they are often portrayed as. Rather denialists are trapped in their denialism. From the denialists' perspective, AIDS is a battle ground to play out a sense of good versus evil, with evil being the government scientists, medical establishment, and drug companies. To suggest otherwise would be to just as easily turn the denialists' inverted world right-side up.

Psychologically, certain people seem predisposed to suspicious thinking, and it seems this may be true of denialism as well. I submit that denialism stems from a conspiracy-theory-prone personality style. We see this in people who appear predisposed to suspiciousness, and these people are vulnerable to anti-establishment propaganda. We know that suspicious people view themselves as the target of wrongdoing and hold persecutory ideas. Suspicious people also tend to be overly independent in their thinking and even in their interpersonal relationships. The source of this independence is of a pervasive unwillingness to trust others. Suspiciousness is also commonly characterized by a fear of homosexuality, or even homophobia. A sense of divisiveness brings the suspicious thinker to carve the world into us and them. The distrust of suspicious-thinking people can reach an extreme to which even indisputable objective evidence to the contrary of their beliefs is dismissed and countered. It is then that suspicion buys into conspiracy theories and the suspicious thinker can be called a denialist.

Why AIDS? Why Now?

It is not surprising that AIDS has attracted the attention of pseudoscientists, conspiracy theorists, and suspicious thinkers. AIDS has always been a hot political issue, embroiled in controversy by its very nature. Much of what fuels denialism stems from the political and cultural heritage of the disease. There is clearly extreme social conservative support for denialism, with prominent conservative web sites offering a home to denialist writings. For example, the *American Journal of Physicians and Surgeons* presents itself as a legitimate scientific journal and offers an outlet for articles on topics with a politically conservative bent. It also provides an outlet for denialist writings and uncritical reviews of denialist books. An affiliated organization, *The Semmelweis Society International*, honored denialists Peter Duesberg and Celia Farber for their exposing the truth about HIV not causing AIDS. Political Libertarians have also jumped to endorse the rights of denialists, particularly with respect to freedom of expression issues, and without apparent consideration of the harm caused by much of denialists' speech. Ignoring and misrepresenting AIDS science does not help anyone. The populations most affected by AIDS are also among the most marginalized, including gay men, racial minorities, drug users, and the inner-city poor – all are favorite targets of the extreme socially conservative right.

The fact that HIV is transmissible between persons also feeds fear, attracting people prone to paranoid thinking. Irrational fears of germs and contagions as well as obsessions with homosexuality and conspiracies are paramount in paranoia. It is no wonder that a widespread sexually transmitted virus that is prevalent in gay communities would attract the interest of the paranoid personality. The AIDS fatigue factor also appears to open the door to denialism. Public health education campaigns have dwindled over time, with new generations not being educated about AIDS. There is also growing complacency in response to HIV/AIDS, especially as HIV infection becomes a medically manageable disease (Appendix A presents a timeline of HIV/AIDS denialism).

The Internet also plays a critical role in the rise of denialism, offering fringe groups access to a global audience. Pseudoscience on the Internet is easily confused with legitimate science. People living with HIV/AIDS often seek answers by searching the Internet. Many denialists attribute their awakening to reading the facts about AIDS on the Internet or in life stories of denialists published online. Among denialists, none is known better than South Africa's former President Thabo Mbeki, who became involved in denialism by surfing the Internet.

Denialism is also at least partly an outgrowth of a more general anti-science and anti-medicine movement. There is public distrust against the US Food and Drug Administration and the pharmaceutical industry. Every time there is a recall of approved medications, as happens all too often, public trust is eroded. Campaigns against teaching evolution in favor of creationism, now referred to as Intelligent Design, remain as commonplace today as ever. Conservative political groups have called the peer-review process into question, further heightening suspicions toward science and medicine.

Scientists are generally good at communicating with each other, but often fail to communicate effectively with the public. Public health agencies also fail to provide useful and accurate science-based information on HIV/AIDS, undoubtedly playing an important role in the rise of denialism. Unfulfilled promises and predictions made by scientists and politicians through press conferences and media interviews also raise suspicions about AIDS science. AIDS pseudoscientists and denialists have seized on failed scientific predictions in making their point that science is a fraud. In some cases, denialists distort predictions, stating them in more certain terms than they were originally intended. In other cases, denialists selectively pick from partially fulfilled predictions to buttress their case.

Table 1.1 summarizes predictions that denialists commonly point to as proof that HIV does not cause AIDS. Denialists ask the question, "With all of the money and all of the attention poured into AIDS research, why have these predictions not panned out?" As shown in the table, most of the predictions

Table 1.1 Predictions in the history of AIDS science, their use by denialists and evidence-based status

Historical prediction	HIV/AID denialist myth	Scientific fact
HIV causes immune deficiency by killing CD4/T-cells.	HIV does not kill cells. HIV=AIDS theory says that HIV programs cells to commit suicide.	HIV does kill CD4/T-cells in the laboratory and in the body. The specific systematic loss of CD4/T-cells only occurs with HIV infection and is the cause of AIDS.
HIV will spread rapidly throughout the heterosexual population.	In 1987, there were predictions that one in five Americans will have AIDS within a decade.	HIV did not spread as originally predicted. We later learned that there are multiple strains of the virus that are spread more easily in different ways. The virus responsible for the US epidemic is more easily spread by anal sex, whereas the African strain is more easily spread by vaginal sex.
AIDS will devastate Africa.	Even the most AIDS-burdened countries of southern Africa continue to experience population growth. The population of Africa has increased more than 300 million since AIDS began.	AIDS has devastated and continues to devastate southern Africa. Countries such as Botswana have experienced negative population growth that can only be explained by HIV/AIDS.
There will soon be a cure for AIDS.	In 1984, Gallo predicted a cure for AIDS in the next 2 years. Now it is likely that a cure will never be found.	HIV/AIDS is becoming medically manageable with antiretroviral medications, and one day, there may be a cure. However, today there remains no cure for HIV/AIDS.
A vaccine to prevent HIV infection will soon be available.	In 1984, Gallo predicted a vaccine in 2 years. All vaccine efforts have failed, and there will not likely be a vaccine because HIV+ people already have HIV antibodies.	Robert Gallo never predicted an HIV vaccine within 2 years, although others in the US Public Health Service did. HIV rapidly mutates, is genetically diverse, and harbors in the

Table 1.1 (continued)

Historical prediction	HIV/AID denialist myth	Scientific fact
		immune system, proving to be evasive to preventive vaccines. There may never be an HIV-preventive vaccine, certainly not for several years to come.
HIV will be spread primarily through sexual transmission, needle stick injuries, and sharing injection drug equipment.	Only 1 in 1000 unprotected sex acts with an HIV+ person transmits HIV, even a constant number of cases could not be sustained in this way. Only 1000 needle stick transmissions have occurred. Injection drug users who use needle exchanges are more likely to test HIV positive than those who do not use clean needles.	The claim that HIV is not spread through vaginal intercourse is false. The modes of HIV transmission identified in the early 1980s have proved correct. Many needle exchange clients are HIV+ because they only started injecting safely after they were infected, in order to protect others from the virus.
HIV will be present in high quantities in people with AIDS.	HIV is proved to barely be found in AIDS patients.	HIV is present in high quantities in people with AIDS. In fact, the highest levels of HIV in the blood occur when a person has developed AIDS.
People who do not have HIV antibodies will not get AIDS.	AIDS does occur in people who do not have HIV antibodies, but they are not classified as AIDS.	There are other causes of immune suppression, such as cancer chemotherapy and malnutrition, but there are no other causes of the selective depletion of CD4 T-cells that results in the syndrome we call AIDS.
AIDS will develop within 5 years of a person getting HIV infected.	A prediction made in the mid-1980s has had to change repeatedly and is now at 10 years. No one really knows, and this	The natural history of HIV in causing AIDS is now known to occur over an average of 10 years, which can be substantially

Table 1.1 (continued)

Historical prediction	HIV/AID denialist myth	Scientific fact
	estimate creates a conundrum when the first AIDS cases among people in their early twenties are considered.	extended with antiretroviral therapy.
AIDS does not discriminate.	AIDS remains contained in risk groups in the United States and Europe – gay men and injection drug users. Mostly men have AIDS in these countries. Even more damning is that different risk groups have different AIDS-defining conditions.	HIV/AIDS occurs in subgroups because of patterns of risk behaviors and networks of people who carry and transmit the virus. Different risk groups get different AIDS-defining conditions simply because of differences in exposure to those other disease-causing agents.
Anti-HIV medications will stop HIV infection.	The annual mortality rate of HIV+ people being treated is much higher than those not treated. People who are treated are much more likely to die of cardiac failure and liver disease than they would have from AIDS.	We remain hopeful that antiretrovirals will one day eradicate HIV from the body. This would be a cure for HIV/AIDS. Today, HIV treatments slow the virus and extend years of life, but the medications do not stop the infection. People with HIV/AIDS are also more likely to die while on treatment because the treatments are typically not started until late in the disease process.
Commercial sex workers will be decimated by AIDS.	Prostitutes are not at risk for AIDS, unless they inject drugs, and there are virtually no clients who have contracted AIDS from a prostitute.	This myth is proved wrong by countless medical studies of sex workers in the United States, Africa, Asia, and elsewhere. Sex workers who have never injected drugs contract HIV and have infected subsequent sex partners.

Note: Failed AIDS predictions adapted from R. Culshaw (2007). *Science Sold Out.*

made by AIDS scientists are supported by subsequent evidence. Some predictions, however, reflect the limited knowledge about AIDS in the 1980s. Still others, particularly predicted cures and vaccines, failed to appreciate the complexity of HIV infection.

Denialism has taken hold as a troublesome social phenomenon. Like its siblings – AIDS stigma, homophobia, and racism – denialism is more than an irritant, more than a handful of rogue scientists, and more than a bunch of crackpots on the Internet. Denialism creates confusion between pseudoscience and science, and between fraud and medicine. Denialism also provides political cover for policy makers, including presidents, whose political and economic interests often outweigh their interests in public health. Unlike most other problems in the fight against AIDS, however, denialism has been neglected by researchers and activists – perhaps because those who follow the denialists are invisible to us. Or perhaps because we have focused on what have seemed like more pressing problems. Or perhaps because the default strategy has been to ignore denialism and hope it will go away – or to believe it has already gone away. Clearly, the strategy of denial in response to denialism has failed.

Who Are the Denialists?

Not surprisingly, there is a list of denialists or "AIDS Rethinkers" posted on the Internet. Over 2700 people listed are described as "Very serious, concerned, and highly educated people from every corner of the globe." The purpose of the list is to rebut those who say that "only a handful of scientists doubt HIV's role in AIDS."[15] What is obvious is that the list of Rethinkers is a definitive directory of denialists. What is not so obvious is that it also serves as a means for denialists to see who has been vetted and cleared for insider communication.

Few on the list actually have any scientific credentials, and those who do are key figures in denialism. In late 2007, there was also a movement among anti-denialists, such as the aidstruth.org group, to verify the names on the list. Anti-denialism activists started contacting people on the list to ask whether they were aware that they were listed as AIDS Rethinkers. These contacts resulted in some listed members becoming outraged and asking to be removed, I suppose by a process of unvetting. Names started being blacked out from the list with the explanation that the "Names removed due to fear and intimidation." I spoke with a retired public health researcher who had coauthored a paper with a denialist and ended up on the list. He told me that he was surprised that he was listed as an AIDS Rethinker and insisted that he be removed, stating that he did not want to be associated with the group. Others threatened to sue Rethinking AIDS if they were not removed. AIDS Rethinkers would have us believe that people are asking for their names to be removed because they are scared of being associated with people who question HIV as the cause of AIDS, victims of a conspiracy to persecute and censor AIDS dissidents.

It is essential to realize that denialism is not a solely US phenomenon. There are denialist groups on every continent, and their work appears in every medium. Televangelists, such as Ken Greene of Greenville South Carolina, see AIDS as the wrath of God placed upon those who sin. Minister Greene has preached about the sins of homosexuality, and he is the founder of African Harvest Ministries, where he claims documented proof that he has cured people of AIDS by performing miracles. In Ethiopia, more than one in four people with HIV/AIDS who are given treatments stop taking their medications because their spiritual leaders have told them to drink holy water instead. There are gay activist groups, most notably the now defunct ACTUP San Francisco, who view AIDS as a product of government conspiracies against the gay community. Denialism has also emerged from deranged and disgruntled university professors who turn to pseudoscience as a platform to gain attention. There are also unscrupulous entrepreneurs who rely on pseudoscience to sell fake cures. There are untrained scientist wannabes for whom denialism is only one facet of a personal mission against the medical establishment. There are also sensationalist journalists and Internet bloggers who sell AIDS denialism as a good conspiracy story. Among denialists are heads of state that have turned away from AIDS science in favor of denialist views. Other heads of state have even invented potions that they claim to cure AIDS (Appendix B provides a brief synopsis or who's who among denialists).

In all of its forms, denialism is inextricably intertwined with AIDS pseudoscience. AIDS pseudoscience propagates denialist myths through unregulated and non-scientific communication outlets, particularly books, magazines, and the Internet, as well as the exploitation of non-peer reviewed avenues within scientific outlets, such as letters to editors and commentaries.

Denialists are not just a few renegade crackpots looking for attention. Internet postings suggest thousands of people to at least question the science behind HIV as the cause of AIDS. There are support groups for people who have tested HIV positive and refute their medical diagnosis. In 2007, there were "AIDS dissident" science conferences held in Paris and Berlin. An online AIDS dissident encyclopedia style web site AIDS Wiki boasts over 70,000 visits, and the Alberta Reappraising AIDS Society web site claims over a million visits. The proliferation of denialist writings through multiple media outlets does more than distract AIDS scientists; it undermines countless efforts to save lives.

Why We Should Care About Denialism

Denialists cause me less concern than people who desperately search for information about AIDS and stumble on their web sites and books. If no one paid attention to the denialists, they would be little more than an amusing blip in the history of AIDS, and I would not have written this book. Unfortunately, denialists are responsible for a significant amount of death and suffering. Faced with a life-threatening illness, people diagnosed with HIV infection will undoubtedly search for hope and cures, with the casual onlooker unable to distinguish between pseudoscience and science, between bogus quackery and genuine medicine. The credibility gap becomes fuzziest in claims found on the Internet, in books, and in the popular press. Pseudoscience also creeps into the mainstream through letters to scientific journals and publication outlets with limited review.

Consider this example of credibility creep in AIDS pseudoscience; it comes from a review of a book by Henry Bauer, a science professor at Virginia Tech University who claims HIV does not exist. Bauer's book *The Origins, Persistence and Failings of HIV/AIDS Theory* claims to prove that HIV cannot cause AIDS. William F. Shughart is the editor of a peer-reviewed professional journal in economics and political science, *Public Choice,* the outlet of the Public Choice Society; Shughart, included the following:

> The epidemiology of AIDS in Africa is different. Its signature diseases there are "not the same as the characteristic AIDS diseases in Europe and North America." As a matter of fact, because diagnosing AIDS in Africa does not require a positive HIV test, "deaths from causes that have beset Africans for a long time" may simply have been reclassified as AIDS-related. Nevertheless, mortality rates from all causes have not risen sharply in Africa. Fear-mongering about an AIDS "epidemic" in Africa plausibly reflects naked self interest: "the world has been generous with help against AIDS while not generous with help against ordinary poverty and malnutrition." Bono, call your office.[16]

Accepting the content of Henry Bauer's book as credible is a mistake that anyone who knows nothing about AIDS could make, I suppose. But the nonsense of this book is readily apparent to anyone with even a basic understanding of the HIV/AIDS epidemic or basic principles of epidemiology. Nevertheless, when a journal editor publishes a positive book review, he creates an impression of credibility for Bauer's ill-conceived thesis.

Ultimately, denialism promotes distrust in the diagnosis and treatment of HIV/AIDS. Why get tested when the results are invalid? Why receive treatment when the virus is harmless? Why earmark more money for treatment programs in Africa when mortality rates there are more or less the same as they have always been? Merely raising these questions refutes AIDS science, fosters a sense of personal denial, and interferes with treatment options and policy decisions. Denialism can cultivate maladaptive and even malignant denial in people who have tested HIV positive. Denialism has influenced people who make policy, teach students, and lecture to the public at large. These are the fundamental harms caused by propagating denialism and the basis for my sense of urgency in writing this book.

Denialism has a definite political dimension. Denialists can influence government policies on HIV testing, HIV prevention, and HIV/AIDS treatment. Policies such as banning people with HIV from entering the United States, prohibiting access to sterile needles and syringes, insisting on abstinence for prevention, banning condoms in prison, and interfering with access to HIV treatments are examples of how denialism has caused unknown amounts of suffering. Denialism can also cut off millions of dollars in resources from much-needed programs. Thousands or tens or hundreds of thousands of people have not gained access to HIV treatments and thousands or tens or hundreds of thousands of babies have needlessly been born with HIV infection – and denialism has helped that failure, that turning away from the truth, happen. To not understand how destructive denialism can be is to have one's head in the sand.

Peter Duesberg and the Origins of HIV/AIDS Denialism

Epidemiology is like a bikini: what is revealed is interesting; what is concealed is crucial.

Peter Duesberg, 1991

Ultimately it comes down to trust. Trusting what you hear. Trusting what you read. Trusting what one world-acclaimed scientist says over another. If denialism did not have a scientifically credible proponent it would never have been considered worthy of attention. But denialism has such a proponent.

Confusion as to whether HIV is the cause of AIDS is traceable to one man, Peter Duesberg. As a scientist, Duesberg appears credible because of his training and his indisputably impressive early career accomplishments.

Duesberg is in fact many things to many people, and opinions about him tend to split into extremes: Is Peter Duesberg an accomplished scientist or a deranged crackpot? Is he a victim of a conspiracy against dissident AIDS scientists or a perpetrator of denialism on a global scale? Has he attracted a cadre of legitimate scientists who share his dissident views or is he a magnet for pseudoscientists and the disaffected and deranged? Is Peter Duesberg a symbol of the routine suppression of truth in modern science or is he merely a bitter man with an axe to grind? The leader of a movement or a cult hero?

Although Peter Duesberg is arguably the most important figure in denialism, he is certainly not alone. One could argue that President Ronald Reagan – who took office in 1981 but did not speak about AIDS until 1987, after nearly 50,000 Americans had been diagnosed with AIDS and more than half had died – was a significant early contributor to the cause of denialism. And the earliest formal expression of denialism did not come from Peter Duesberg but from Casper Schmidt, who responded to early AIDS science in a paper called "The Group-Fantasy Origins of AIDS." Schmidt, a well known gay psychiatrist in New York stated in 1984 that AIDS was an "epidemic hysteria" in which individuals were acting out "social conflicts." Schmidt, after stating that AIDS was the result of conservative sexual repression and moral condemnation, wrote this in an academic journal in 1984:

> According to this interpretation, the viral etiology which is subscribed to by many should be seen as part of the unconscious group delusion of a poison threat. The evidence presented so far supports the view that the virus which has been discovered (LAV/HTLV-III) is probably just another opportunistic infection, and plays, if at all, only a late role in the causal chain of AIDS. As in other epidemics, the poison which "causes" the disorder is assumed to originate from outside the country.[1]

Casper Schmidt died of AIDS in 1994.

But if Schmidt was an earlier practitioner of denialism, and Reagan, in his silence, was effective at keeping the issue of AIDS out of the public's consciousness, Peter Duesburg remains the individual who has done the most damage because he has given denialism its air of scientific legitimacy, which to this day helps keep it alive. What makes Duesberg unique in the world of denialism are his scientific credentials. The credibility that Duesberg gained from the very peers he turned on is precisely what gives him voice. Duesberg infuriated the scientific establishment by his betrayal of objectivity and abandonment of the rules of science, but to understand the origins of HIV/AIDS denialism and its continuing power today, it is necessary to explore his world.

Who Is Peter Duesberg?

Peter Duesberg was born in Munster, Germany in 1936 and was educated at the Universities of Wurtzberg, Frankfurt, and Munich as well as the University of Basel in Switzerland. Both of his parents were physicians with his father serving as a doctor in the German army during Second World War. Duesberg received his doctorate degree in chemistry from the University of Frankfurt in 1963 and has been on the faculty of the University of California, Berkeley, since 1964, achieving the rank of Full Professor in the Department of Molecular and Cell Biology. By all accounts, Duesberg possesses a brilliant mind.

His early research focused on the genetic bases of cancer. He was among the first scientists to isolate cancer-causing genes and cancer-related retroviruses – viruses that integrate their genetic material (RNA) into the genetic make up of cells (DNA) to replicate themselves. Duesberg's discoveries clearly led to greater understanding of the role that genetics plays in cancer. He worked with other Berkeley scientists, including acclaimed molecular biologist G. Steve Martin, to discover the first cancer-causing genes – oncogenes. The Berkeley Group was among the first to demonstrate that retroviruses carry oncogenes that transform normal cells into deadly cancer cells. Understanding the genetics of cancer brought about new and sophisticated technologies that have become critical in cancer prevention and treatment. Peter Duesberg's work in cancer also led to his election to the National Academy of Sciences in 1986. The citation for his membership to the Academy reads:

> The first true oncogene, src, was identified and mapped by Duesberg. He also chemically mapped the entire viral genome and then duplicated these feats for three major mouse sarcoma viruses and some half-dozen avian sarcoma and leukemia viruses.[2]

Throughout the 1970s and 1980s, Duesberg had his own highly regarded and productive basic sciences lab at Berkeley. The National Cancer Institute (NCI), one of the major branches of the National Institutes of Health (NIH), was the primary source of his research funding. In 1986, he received the rare honor of an Outstanding Investigator Research Grant from the NIH. Duesberg's advances in cancer science were indisputably leading edge. He was among a small handful of elite biomedical researchers on the forefront of unraveling the mysteries of cancer.

The role of oncogenes in causing cancer follows the same logic as other inherited characteristics. Our DNA contains the blueprint that determines all of our physical traits. In the case of oncogenes, some of us are born with a genetic tendency toward developing a specific cancer. Oncogenes explain why certain cancers run in families, and identifying oncogenes has led to genetic tests that have aided prevention, early detection, and treatment of many types of cancers. The link between retroviruses and oncogenes was also

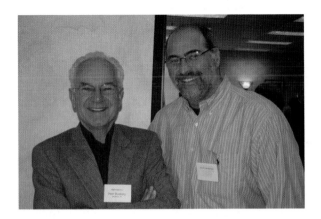

Photo 2.1 Meeting Peter Duesberg, Oakland California, February 2008

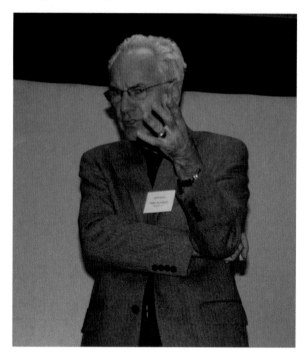

Photo 2.2 Peter Duesberg lectures on Aneuploidy, Oakland California, February 2008

becoming apparent, such as in the case of some types of leukemia, where retroviruses insert oncogenes into our genetic material (DNA) in our cells that then mutate and develop cancer.

Having done much of the early important work on the genetics of cancer, and having played a key role in pointing cancer research in a new direction, Peter Duesberg made what appears to be a radical shift in his thinking in the early 1980s. To put it simply, he changed his mind about the cause of cancer. During this time, he published papers in the distinguished journals *Nature* and *Science* in which he completely dismissed the role of retroviruses and oncogenes in causing cancer. He refuted his own work on retroviruses and rejected the concept of oncogenes being sufficient to cause cancer. Duesberg also launched a series of criticisms of other cancer researchers who had embraced his work on oncogenes as the cause of cancer, including prominent and influential researchers such as J. Michael Bishop and Harold Varmus, whose work on oncogenes – just across the bay, at the University of California San Francisco – led to a Nobel Prize in 1989. Bishop and Varmus demonstrated that genes called non-cancer-causing proto-oncogenes mutate to defective oncogenes that occur in many organisms, including humans.

Duesberg took a radically different path, concluding that retroviruses were virtually harmless and incapable of causing cancer. In 1987 he stated, "Since the viruses associated with all human tumors and most natural tumors of animals are latent and frequently defective, it is difficult to justify the claims that these viruses play any causative role in tumorigenesis."[3] Remarkably, the claim that viruses play a causative role in developing tumors was his very own, made just a few years earlier. But the change in position was starkly clear, and Duesberg did not back down from it. He outright rejects the fact that genes mutate to cause cancer. To this day, he dismisses the idea that a retrovirus can cause cancer, and in fact doubts whether any virus can cause any cancer. He apparently even rejects the indisputable link between Human Papillomavirus (HPV) and cervical cancer.

Why would this distinguished scientist, after first having discovered one of the most promising avenues for cancer research, abandon his ideas, bringing what was a highly productive line of research to a grinding halt? Why would he turn from discoverer to dissident? It is a puzzle worth considering.

Duesberg shifted his view of cancer toward a theory proposed by the German scientist Theodor Boveri (1862–1915), who in 1914 proposed that chromosomal mutations, not gene mutations, collectively called Aneuploidy are the cause of cancer. Specifically, Aneuploidy is the name given to cells that develop an abnormal number of chromosomes. Nearly all cells in the human body contain 23 pairs of chromosomes, or 46 in total. Genes, which contain our DNA code, in turn make up our chromosomes. During reproductive division, errors can result in cells with too many, and others with too few, chromosomes. Having an abnormal number of chromosomes usually results in cell death. However, when cells that have an abnormal number of chromosomes, or Aneuploidy, survive they divide and grow with significant detrimental consequences. In genetic theories of cancer, mutated oncogenes trigger rampant abnormal growth of cells, including Aneuploidy. In opposition to the mainstream that he helped to establish, Duesberg theorizes that oncogenes are not the cause of cancerous growth; they are merely passengers that just happen to be present. What is critical here is that Duesberg extends his more general view of retroviruses and oncogenes to explain AIDS.

In addition to mutated oncogenes causing Aneuploidy, the defect can also result from exposure to environmental toxins including radiation, chemicals, and other carcinogens. Duesberg takes the extreme position that Aneuploidy is not the *effect* of cancer, but rather the opposite; and that Aneuploidy resulting from environmental carcinogens is the sole cause of *all* cancers. In Duesberg's approach, the oncogenes he once helped discover become irrelevant passengers of no consequence, as shown in Figs. 2.1 and 2.2.

Duesberg ultimately concluded that retroviruses and the genetic material they carry, including oncogenes, cannot cause disease. Duesberg switched his

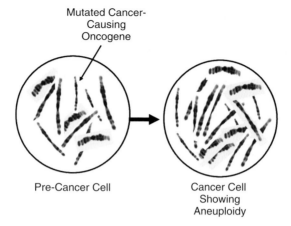

Fig. 2.1 The genetic theory of cancer, in which mutated oncogenes cause cancerous cell growth resulting in an abnormal number of chromosomes called Aneuploidy

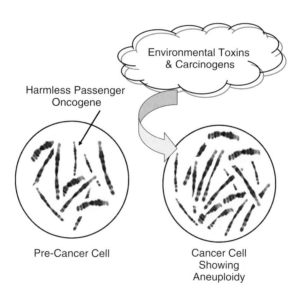

Fig. 2.2 Peter Duesberg's theory of cancer, in which oncogenes are irrelevant passengers, while environmental carcinogens cause Aneuploidy, which in turn results in cancerous cell growth

thinking from a genetic basis for cancer (where oncogenes set in motion the processes that lead to the disease) to an environmental basis (where toxins cause Aneuploidy, which in turn causes the disease). He then extended this view to explain AIDS.

To understand Duesberg's theory about what causes AIDS, it is best to begin with an account of how our understanding of AIDS developed in the late twentieth century, as the epidemic spread. By the late 1980s, scientists were beginning to understand that as a retrovirus, HIV enters specifically targeted cells, the T-Helper Lymphocytes, by attaching to a molecule called CD4 on their cell membranes. The retrovirus transfers its genetic material (RNA) into the cell, where it integrates with the cell's DNA to take control and replicate itself. Enzymes such as reverse transcriptase, protease, and integrase are critical to the HIV replication process (and later became the target of antiretroviral drugs). But in a 1987 article in the journal *Cancer Research*, Duesberg suggested that retroviruses might be harmless tag-alongs, mere passengers, that are insufficient to cause disease – either cancer or AIDS. As shown in Figs. 2.3 and 2.4, Duesberg's theory of AIDS carries the same conceptual basis as his theory of cancer, where genetics are irrelevant and human-made conditions are the cause of disease. The questions he raised about whether retroviruses can cause AIDS were crystallized as definitive statements in subsequent articles in prestigious scientific journals, defining Duesberg as the most visible dissident AIDS scientist in the world, despite his never actually doing any work on HIV or AIDS.

In 1993, Duesberg's research funding from NIH ended, essentially knocking him into the minor leagues of biomedical science. Although Duesberg maintains his own privately funded laboratory at the University of California Berkeley, he is not a part of The Cancer Research Laboratory at the university. He has tried to obtain research funding from the NIH more than 20 times since 1993, but without success. Journalist Celia Farber describes Duesberg's laboratory in the Donner Building, which is set in a beautiful area of the wooded Berkeley campus, as a modest space with few resources. He has only

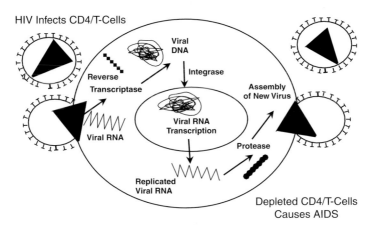

Fig. 2.3 The established description of how HIV infects CD4/T-Helper cells to cause AIDS

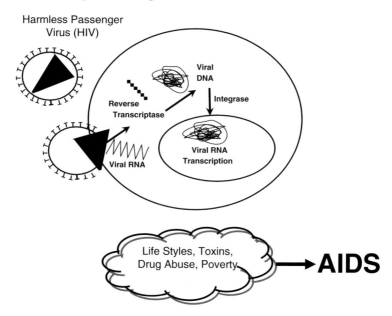

Fig. 2.4 Peter Duesberg's theory of AIDS where HIV is an irrelevant passenger virus and environmental toxins and contaminants cause AIDS

a couple lab technicians and is funded by a private donor who also has HIV/AIDS denialist interests. By his own account, Duesberg describes his downward turn as follows:

> I had all the students I wanted. I had all the lab space I needed. I got all the grants awarded. I was elected to the National Academy. I became California Scientist of the Year. All my papers were published. I could do no wrong. Almost, professionally, that is, until I started questioning the claim that HIV or the hypothesis that HIV is the cause of AIDS. Then everything changed.[4]

Duesberg attributes his professional demise to his being an AIDS dissident. Many other accounts of the academic career of Peter Duesberg portray the same image. However, it is important to note that he publicly began questioning HIV as the cause of AIDS at the same time that he refutes the idea that oncogenes cause cancer. It would appear, then, that abandoning oncogenes (and taking up Aneuploidy) was the defining moment for Duesberg. Searching the National Library of Medicine for the term "oncogene" retrieves over 130,000 scientific references, whereas "aneuploidy cancer" retrieves just over 8,000 references. A search of the same terms in the NIH grants database shows that the National Cancer Institute has awarded over 460 grants to study oncogenes whereas fewer than 40 grants have been awarded to investigate

Aneuploidy. Unless there is a conspiracy against the entire idea of Aneuploidy as the cause of cancer, which Duesberg and his followers may very well claim, it is apparent that Duesberg departed from studying oncogenes for the less promising avenue of Aneuploidy.

I attended Duesberg and David Rasnick's conference on Aneuploidy and cancer in 2008 to get a sense of what this was all about. Two legitimate cancer researchers that I spoke with felt uneasy coming to the conference, which was attended by about 40 people and held in the meeting room of a small Oakland hotel. They felt that Aneuploidy was an important feature of cancer, although not necessarily the cause of cancer. One of the researchers told me of how she was experiencing difficulty getting her own NIH grant on chromosomal aspects of cancer funded. She had no prior association with Duesberg and was not under any impression that there was a conspiracy against her work, although the dominant views on genetics as a cause of cancer may have been an issue. She seemed understandably frustrated, but was not calling for an international investigation into the corruption of peer review.

Peter Duesberg's scientific reputation is so damaged that when the magazine *Scientific American* published his article "Chromosomal Chaos" on Aneuploidy and cancer the Editors included the following disclaimer:

> Editors' note: The author, Peter Duesberg, a pioneering virologist, may be well known to readers for his assertion that HIV is not the cause of AIDS. The biomedical community has roundly rebutted that claim many times. Duesberg's ideas about chromosomal abnormality as a root cause for cancer, in contrast, are controversial but are being actively investigated by mainstream science. We have therefore asked Duesberg to explain that work here. This article is in no sense an endorsement by *Scientific American* of his AIDS theories.[5]

A fundamental question that was suggested by Celia Farber is, "Did the NIH de-fund Peter Duesberg's research because of his views on AIDS?" The conclusion that Duesberg has been excluded from NIH grant funding is propagated by conservative journalists such as Tom Bethell, as reported by Steven Milloy for Fox News in 2005:

> Bethell points out that the man who "rediscovered" the old work on Aneuploidy is controversial University of California-Berkeley researcher and National Academy of Sciences member Peter Duesberg, who famously had his grants from the National Institutes of Health cut off for being critical of the direction of AIDS research in the late-1980s. Duesberg still isn't getting any NIH money even though his Aneuploidy idea has survived early challenges, according to Bethell's article, and the older notions of cancer development are going nowhere fast.[6]

Contrary to journalistic accounts, Duesberg was not "de-funded" by the NIH. All research grants come to an end, and Duesberg's grant ended in 1991. Also, he did not "lose" funding for AIDS because he was never funded to do

AIDS research. Rather, it was his cancer research that ended. His final grants from the National Cancer Institute were titled "Structural and Replication of Rous Sarcoma and Influenza" and "Molecular and Genetics Analyses of RNA Tumor viruses." And his most prestigious research grant was titled "Retro-viral Oncogenes and Cellular Proto-Oncogenes." Peter Duesberg was success-ful in receiving very competitive research grants from the NIH when he was researching oncogenes. As I noted earlier, Aneuploidy can hardly be con-sidered a hot new avenue in cancer research.

In 1993, Duesberg did apply for a grant from the National Institute of Drug Abuse entitled "Animal tests of the AIDS risks of nitrite inhalants." The grant was not funded, and its resubmission received the recommendation that "No Further Consideration be Given to this Application," meaning that is could not be submitted again – the fate of a grant application that cannot be improved with revisions. Duesberg and his supporters maintain that he is the victim of a conspiracy against him for speaking out against the theory that HIV causes AIDS – the theory championed by his arch-rival Robert Gallo.

Peter Duesberg and Robert Gallo

It is virtually impossible to understand Duesberg's involvement in AIDS without examining his relationship with Robert Gallo. The ties between Duesberg and Gallo date back well before the AIDS era, when both scientists were supported by the National Cancer Institute and both were studying retroviruses as potential causes of cancer. Gallo has numerous scientific contributions to his credit, including discovering the retroviruses that cause certain types of leukemia. He is best known, though, as the co-discoverer of the retrovirus later named HIV. The history of HIV's discovery, its rediscovery, and ultimately its co-discovery by Gallo and French scientist Luc Montagnier in 1984, is a story told countless times by all parties involved. The race to find what was mysteriously killing young men and women was indeed newsworthy; it was so widely anticipated as breaking news that its was leaked to the press prior to the publication of the research articles. There were headlines around the globe, and Gallo correctly predicted that the discovery of the virus would lead to a test to screen donated blood and save thousands of lives.

In 1984, Duesberg was not concerned with finding the cause of AIDS. However, the discovery by Gallo and Montagnier, and perhaps the attendant publicity, may have shaped his decision to abandon retroviruses and onco-genes as a cause of cancer and in doing so also refuting HIV as the cause of

AIDS. The relationship between Duesberg and Gallo has played out in many places. Gallo dedicates several pages of his book *Virus Hunting* to directly confronting Duesberg, and Duesberg references Gallo throughout his manifesto *Rethinking the AIDS Virus.* As I noted above, Gallo had previously discovered the retrovirus that causes a certain type of leukemia, namely human T-cell lymphotropic virus type-1 or HTLV-I. Discovering this virus led to new tests and new treatments for leukemia – good research, even great work, that doubtless saved lives. A second retrovirus, HTLV-II shares similar genetic characteristics with HTLV-I, but is less common and not linked to disease. Gallo identified the retrovirus that causes AIDS and initially named it HTLV-III, and later renamed it HIV. There was great controversy regarding whether Gallo discovered the virus and ultimately it was determined that the virus was discovered by his French counterparts. Gallo has made numerous other important discoveries, including his discovery in 1995 that chemokines, a class of naturally occurring compounds, can block HIV and halt its progression of AIDS. The controversy over the discovery of HIV most likely cost Gallo a Nobel Prize; but he was and will be for all time, the co-discoverer of the virus that causes AIDS, and that goes beyond headlines to a place in history.

As scientists working in the same field and on the same problem, Duesberg and Gallo knew each other well. A famous quote of Gallo introducing Duesberg at a meeting held at the National Cancer Institute in 1984, near the time that Gallo first announced the discovery of HIV, speaks volumes about the relationship between the two men. Having spent a couple days sitting next to Duesberg at his Aneuploidy conference, it is my impression that the following historical quote captures the very essence of the man. After running through several of Duesberg's achievements, Gallo ended by saying:

> These are some of Peter's contributions. There are many more. However, there are things about him that stand out as much as his science. Peter Duesberg is a man of extraordinary energy, unusual honesty, enormous sense of humor, and a rare critical sense. This critical sense often makes us look twice, then a third time, at a conclusion many of us believed to be foregone. However, his critiques are sometimes a major problem for the casual observer. When is he truly debating? When is he only being the devil's advocate? When is he being the devil himself? The casual observer is also often at a loss to determine which of the many weapons he possesses he is using. Peter, it is hard for us to tell when you are using your machine gun or your slingshot, or simply exercising your vocal cords. In any event you are an extraordinary scientist, a man who makes life more interesting and pleasurable to many of us: and it is my good fortune to know you as a friend.[7]

Soon after this meeting, Gallo announced his discovering the retrovirus that causes AIDS. Duesberg and Gallo soon became embroiled in their own controversy regarding whether HIV causes AIDS. Their relationship descended into personal attacks that persisted throughout the 1990s, playing out in magazine articles, interviews, and books. A typical example of a Duesberg attack on Gallo and Luc Montagnier, which at once captures his sharp wit and his bitterness, occurs in his *Inventing the AIDS Virus*:

> Gallo and Montagnier probably assumed HIV is new because it was newly discovered by them. But since the technology used to detect HIV is just as new as the discovery of HIV, there is another interpretation: Gallo and Montagnier discovered a previously unknown old virus with a new technique. Their claim that HIV is new is just as naïve as the claim of an astronomer that a previously unknown star is new because it became detectable with a new telescope. . ... Indeed, Gallo and Montagnier's reasoning fits their narrow expertise exactly. Two leading retrovirologists agreeing on a retrovirus as the cause of AIDS and ignoring all competing retroviral and non-retroviral explanations. And for the leaders, ignorance is bliss.[8]

Ultimately, Duesberg claimed that his being critical of Gallo and the NIH cost him his career. In a 1993 talk, he gave for University of California Berkeley Alumni, Duesberg stated:

> Now, if you were to decide what AIDS is caused by, you should ask first. . .we should have asked at the beginning, is AIDS actually an infectious disease? Even the CDC considered lifestyle interpretations until the famous Gallo-Heckler press conference. Because that came from the NIH, it was binding to all public health institutes in the country, to the CDC, to the National Institute of Drug Abuse, and to all recipients of research grants, which means everybody who is doing research in the free state universities in this country. Like it or not, they all depend on Robert Gallo, Sam Broder, and Anthony Fauci for their grants, because otherwise their machines would stop grinding because these universities could never pay for the equipment that we need in the laboratory. It all comes from the central government. We have totalitarian science directed entirely from Washington in hypothetically free universities. You can survive with tenure but you certainly cannot run a centrifuge or pay your graduate students or write a paper if you don't have a government grant.[9]

For Gallo's part, there is no mistaking that Duesberg gets under his skin. There are countless examples of Gallo's frustration. In an interview with Anthony Liversidge for *Spin* magazine in 1988, Gallo responded to this question, "But Duesberg points out that only very low levels of viral RNA have been detected in AIDS antibody-positive blood samples, and that sick AIDS patients have no measurable amount of virus in the blood?," stating:

> Low levels? He does not know what he is talking about. He is quoting our data that the virus doesn't infect a number of cells. Cock and horse shit. Baloney. He misinterprets the experiments we published. The virus doesn't infect only a small number of cells. It infects a lot of cells. It is only expressed at one time in a small

number of cells. [This is] so silly it defies belief. It's a waste of time. You can keep it going in the popular press and such nonsense can go on forever. Doesn't make any sense to respond to it. No thinking scientist involved in the problem knows anything else but that there is one single cause of AIDS, period. [10]

The bickering goes on to this day. Back and forth, we see Duesberg taunting Gallo and Gallo discrediting Duesberg. The exchanges are personal and bear no resemblance to a scientific debate. One has to ask whether Duesberg is simply motivated to question HIV causing AIDS to irritate Gallo, or to repay him for his fame and good fortune. Does Duesberg even really care about AIDS? After all, he has never done any work with HIV or AIDS. Is Duesberg merely aiming to gain attention, or is it his nature to take extreme views against any mainstream science? Is Duesberg serious when he thanks Gallo in the acknowledgements section of the very 1987 article where he claims that HIV does not cause AIDS? I believe that thanking Gallo for his "discussions" in the acknowledgements section of his article in which he questions HIV as the cause of AIDS tells us as much about Duesberg's animosity as it does his views on AIDS.

Beyond the words of Duesberg himself, much of denialism directs anger toward Gallo. As the most visible AIDS scientist in the world, Gallo symbolizes the denialists' image of the scientific establishment, perhaps in the process becoming more of a symbol than a scientist. Today, there are thousands if not tens of thousands of AIDS scientists. Yet only a few receive the kind of attention Gallo got. From the start, in his own early press interactions as well as his portrayal in popular AIDS stories – most notably Randy Shilts' classic book turned movie *And the Band Played On* – Gallo has been and remains a lightning rod. Randy Shilts portrays Gallo as a competitive, non-cooperative and ego-driven scientist: Shilts wrote, "Gallo also worried that the French would be proved right, and he would not get credit for discovering the AIDS agent."[11] In any event, Gallo remains for many the AIDS hero scientist you love to hate.

And the denialists, needing an establishment AIDS hero to pull down, have not missed a chance to get on the bandwagon. Shilts' detailed account of the early days of AIDS is the closest thing we have to an historical archive of the disease. Denialists, however, often misuse or reinvent history as part of building their case against AIDS science. Similar to how AIDS science is morphed into pseudoscience, AIDS history is reframed. Anthony Brink, a South African lawyer turned denialist offers an example of how history can be corrupted in the service of discrediting Gallo:

We speak of Robert Gallo, who told the worried world at a press conference convened by the US Health Department on 23 April 1984, before the publication of any paper for his fellows to assess, that he'd discovered the cause, a virus he said, of the poor health that a narrow subset of gay men with ruinous lifestyles were experiencing – later christened, in a flourish of conceptual surplusage, the Acquired Immune Deficiency Syndrome. Having sneaked through a patent application on the blood test he'd devised for his claimed viral culprit ahead of the previously lodged French one, thus guaranteeing him a fortune in royalties, Gallo went on to publish four papers in *Science* two weeks later. Then the trouble started, an exuberant international disputation over who stole the fake diamonds.[12]

The fixation of denialists on Robert Gallo reflects their greater concern with media attention and personalities than with science. The importance of Gallo in the history of discovering HIV as the cause of AIDS is undeniable, but denialism refutes science conducted by thousands of researchers, most who have never met Gallo, let alone worked with him. Gallo, for the denialists, is a convenient stand-in, and icon, of all they believe is wrong with established AIDS science and medicine.

Duesberg on AIDS

Peter Duesberg's claim that retroviruses such as HTLV-1 cannot cause cancer or any other disease required him to offer an alternative explanation for the cause of AIDS. Because Duesberg does not dispute the existence of either HIV or AIDS, the question he must answer is, "If not HIV, then what causes AIDS?" Duesberg is a theorist when it comes to AIDS because, as mentioned earlier, he has never done any research of his own on HIV. He states that HIV is harmless and a myriad of environmental hazards are the actual causes of AIDS. In the early 1980s, at the beginning of public awareness of the AIDS crisis, people diagnosed with AIDS typically had histories of using addictive drugs. In addition, gay men diagnosed with AIDS had used inhalants (e.g., poppers) in connection with their sexual experiences. Peter Duesberg claimed and still claims that the drugs themselves cause AIDS. In the early 1980s, others agreed.

Over the years, every scientist accepted that HIV was the cause of AIDS, but Duesberg holds to the theory that drugs cause AIDS. Why? Duesberg had made clear in 1987 his belief that retroviruses do not cause cancer and, by extension, that HIV does not cause AIDS. Environmental toxins cause the chromosome abnormalities seen in Aneuploidy, Duesberg's theoretical cause of cancer, and illicit drugs cause the immune dysfunction labeled AIDS. What about people with AIDS who do not use illicit drugs? His reply is that AZT and other chemicals used to treat HIV actually cause AIDS. And what of those people who had AIDS before AZT was approved and had never used drugs? He says there are no such people. What about hemophiliacs and blood transfusion recipients who have never used drugs or been treated with AZT? Duesberg claims that hemophiliacs develop AIDS from contaminated blood clotting factors. What about Africa, where AIDS kills millions and there is no widespread drug use or AZT? Duesberg claims that AIDS in Africa has existed long before there was an HIV test, and that many old diseases result from malnutrition, contaminated drinking water, and poor sanitation; in a word, poverty.

Duesberg's earliest arguments that HIV cannot possibly cause AIDS have remained unchanged. He asserts that AIDS is a cluster of old diseases that result from immune dysfunction that a harmless retrovirus simply cannot cause. He centers his argument on seven basic principles:

- HIV is a harmless retrovirus that does not and cannot cause AIDS.
- HIV is present as a harmless passenger virus in some people who develop AIDS. Nevertheless, the virus is benign – an innocent bystander.
- Lifestyles cause AIDS; in particular lifestyles that expose a person to environmental assaults on the immune system.
- HIV does not fulfill the time-honored laws of biology, or Koch's Principles, that define infectious diseases. German bacteriologist Robert Koch delineated the criteria to consider a bacterium as a cause of disease, namely isolating the agent from people with the disease and seeing whether others subsequently exposed also develop the disease.
- A person infected with HIV does not necessarily develop AIDS.
- AZT and other HIV treatments are toxic and can cause AIDS.
- AIDS in Africa is an old condition caused by poverty, and only made worse by AZT and other drugs used to treat HIV.

Duesberg's explanation for AIDS is actually far more complex and convoluted than how HIV actually causes AIDS, as illustrated in Fig. 2.5. For Duesberg, HIV infection may or may not occur at all in people who have AIDS. HIV is inconsequential and is only sometimes present in people who develop AIDS. Which cause of AIDS we are talking about depends on where you live as well as your lifestyle? For Gay men, drug use causes AIDS. For Gay men who do not use drugs, HIV medications cause AIDS. In Africa, malnutrition causes AIDS. If you are a wealthy African, AZT causes AIDS. If you are a Hemophiliac, treatments for hemophilia cause AIDS. No research has ever even suggested the Duesbergian view of AIDS is true.

Contrary to the Duesbergian theory of AIDS, there is the established description of how HIV causes AIDS. Built from thousands of clinical and laboratory studies the schematic illustration of how HIV causes AIDS is shown in Fig. 2.6. HIV enters the body through direct contact with blood or sexual fluids infected with the virus. Initial infection sets in and the body reacts by

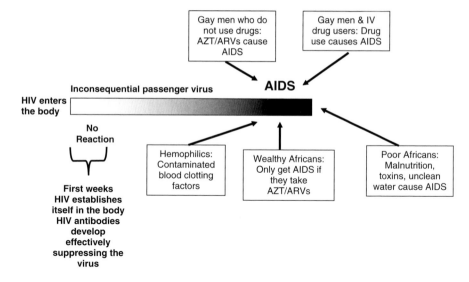

Fig. 2.5 The Duesbergian theory for how multiple external causes of immune suppression result in AIDS. Note: ARVs = antiretroviral medications

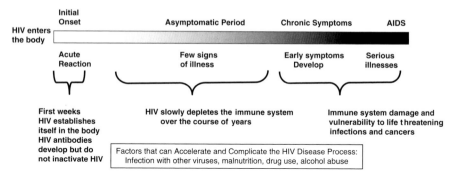

Fig. 2.6 Established model for how HIV depletes the immune system and causes AIDS

producing antibodies against HIV. The virus goes through a latency period, activated later to kill immune cells – specifically CD4 (T-cells). After years of infection, the immune system ultimately collapses and the person develops AIDS, making them vulnerable to infections and cancers. Antiretroviral therapies slow the HIV disease process by suppressing HIV's ability to replicate itself. However, factors that stimulate HIV or run down the immune system, such as poverty and drug abuse, can accelerate HIV disease.

Figure 2.7 details the relationship between HIV infection, CD4/T-Helper cells, and AIDS. In the very first weeks of HIV infection, there is rapid

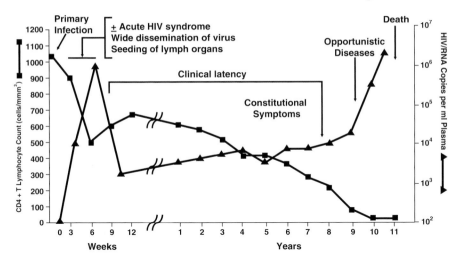

Fig. 2.7 The relationships between HIV concentrations in blood and loss of CD4/T-Helper cells in causing AIDS. Adapted from original sources: http://www.niaid.nih.gov/publications/hivaids/all.htm and Fauci, A., Pantaleo, D., Stanley S., Weismann, D. (1996). Annals of Internal Medicine, volume 124, page 6754

accumulation of HIV in the blood plasma resulting from a high rate of HIV replication without an immediate immune suppressive response. During the acute HIV syndrome, HIV increases (viral load or viremia) along with a rapid decline in CD4/T-Helper cells. The immune system mounts a response that suppresses the amount of virus in the blood and allows a partial rebound in CD4/T-Helper cells. Immune cells and the lymphoid organs harbor HIV, where it depletes the immune system of CD4/T-Helper cells. The process of disrupting and ultimately destroying the immune system takes years. Once CD4/T-Helper cells decline to levels that interfere with their command and control of the immune system, symptoms of late HIV infection emerge, where the person is susceptible to infectious diseases. In the late stages of HIV disease, as many as 10 years after infection with HIV, the immune system becomes depleted and HIV replicates itself at a rapid rate, causing the collapse of the immune system and vulnerability to a myriad of life-threatening opportunistic diseases we call AIDS. Over 130,000 research articles accessed from the National Library of Medicine describe the HIV disease process.

HIV causes havoc in the immune system by selectively infecting the very cells that we rely on to protect us from viruses, specifically CD4/T-Helper lymphocytes. Think of your immune system as your body's army against disease and your CD4/T-Helper cells are that army's generals. These cells orchestrate the multiple components of the immune system to fight disease by sending signals to mount a coordinated immune response. HIV, like all viruses, consists of a small amount of genetic material protected by a protein coat or envelope. In the case of HIV and other retroviruses, the genetic material is RNA. How HIV infects CD4/T-Helper cells to take over the cell's machinery is depicted in Fig. 2.3. The remarkably few genes that make up HIV's genetic material are involved in producing and interacting with over 270 known proteins that are themselves involved in numerous cell functions. At once, HIV is both amazingly simple and devastatingly complex. HIV is a survivor of the immune system because it infects the cells of that very system. HIV is highly adaptive, mutating when pressured by forces in its environment, such as antiretroviral medications, resulting in a great genetic diversity of the virus. It is this genetic diversity and adaptive mutating that has doomed every effort thus far to develop a preventive HIV vaccine.

No basic science or clinical studies show drug abuse, malnutrition, or poverty as the cause of systematic decline in CD4/T-Helper cells that ultimately causes AIDS. To support his conclusion that chemicals, toxins,

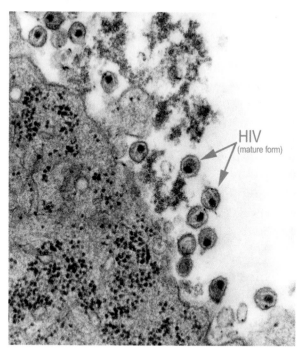

Photo 2.3 Highly magnified transmission electron micrographic (TEM) image of mature forms of the human immunodeficiency virus (HIV) in a tissue sample under investigation. Source: Centers for Disease Control and Prevention, http://phil.cdc.gov/phil/details.asp

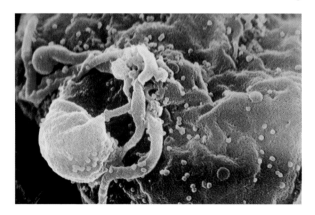

Photo 2.4 Scanning electron micrograph of HIV-1 budding from cultured lymphocyte. See PHIL 1197 for a black and white view of this image. Source: Centers for Disease Control and Prevention, http://phil.cdc.gov/phil/details.asp

and medications cause AIDS, Duesberg relies on trends in population statistics. He compares AIDS cases with drug abuse statistics, claiming that increases in AIDS in the United States, Canada and Europe coincide with increases in drug abuse. Likewise, decreases in AIDS follow trends in decreases in drug abuse. Duesberg's case is, however, highly selective, examining only some drugs some of the time. Duesberg ignores the fact that AIDS declines everywhere in the world when antiretroviral medications become available. In addition, population-level trends do not offer the best evidence for determining the cause of disease. Again, there is no clinical evidence that even the heaviest drug abuse can cause the type and degree of immune system damage that defines AIDS. In fact, there is strong evidence to the exact contrary. Research that has followed large groups of people over long periods of time have shown that those who are HIV positive suffer loss of CD4/T-Helper cells resulting in AIDS, while those who use heavy drugs, including inhalers such as poppers, do not demonstrate loss of CD4/T-Helper cells unless they have HIV. As recently as 2007, researchers studying a large cohort people showed that recreational drug use does not devastate the immune system and that only people who are infected with HIV develop AIDS.[13] The evidence against a drug theory of AIDS could not be any more compelling.

The inconsistencies are even greater for AIDS in Africa. There is no evidence to support Duesberg's claim that malnutrition and contaminated drinking water cause AIDS. Even the most severe poverty does not cause the immune system to collapse as it does in AIDS. Malnutrition is surely the cause of poor health and malnourished people can die of dehydration and starvation. Poverty does not however cause AIDS. Duesberg cannot explain why AIDS has increased rapidly in South Africa, where standards of living

Table 2.1 Poverty indicators and AIDS deaths for 10 developing countries

Country	Estimate of people living on $2 a day or less (%)	Infant mortality rate (per 1000 live births)	Deaths due to AIDS
Bangladesh	82	62.6	Less than 500
Burkina Faso	81	97.6	12,000
Burundi	89	69.2	13,000
Gambia	82	72	1,300
Laos	73	85.2	Less than 100
Mali	90	116.7	11,000
Nepal	83	66.9	5,100
Niger	85	121.6	7,600
Sierra Leon	75	143.6	4,600
South Africa	34	59	320,000

Sources: Poverty and AIDS death statistics from 2006 UNAIDS Global AIDS report, infant mortality statistics from 2005 United Nations poverty index.

have dramatically improved. He also cannot explain the country level disconnect between poverty and AIDS. Table 2.1 shows 10 of the most impoverished countries in the world and the percent of their populations with AIDS. It is easy to see that poverty does not directly coincide with AIDS. For example, Bangladesh has far greater poverty than most countries in the world, and yet there are few cases of AIDS there. Even within Africa, some of the poorest countries – such as Burkina Faso, Gambia, and Mali – are those with the lowest rates of AIDS. If poverty, malnutrition, and unclean water cause AIDS, why does Laos have so little AIDS and South Africa so much? How is it that the rates of people who test HIV positive do parallel the AIDS cases whereas poverty does not? Contrary to Duesberg's theory of AIDS, where there is greater HIV there is more AIDS and where HIV is not prevalent, AIDS cases are low.

Duesberg is also unable to explain the AIDS epidemic among children. In fact, Duesberg has claimed that there is no AIDS epidemic among children. Despite that exceedingly dubious statement, the World Health Organization reports that more than half of a million children in the world were living with HIV/AIDS in 2006, and over 380,000 children died of AIDS in that year. In Zimbabwe alone, nearly 6 percent of orphans to AIDS (both parents died of HIV/AIDS) are HIV positive, almost double the number of non-orphaned children.

Duesberg also makes the preposterous claim that there has never been an AIDS epidemic among prostitutes (commercial sex workers). Unfortunately, he does not offer a basis for this conclusion. Numerous studies report high-rates of HIV infection and correspondingly high-rates of AIDS and death among commercial sex workers. One study conducted in six US cities in the early days of AIDS examined nearly 1,400 female sex workers and found that 12% were HIV positive. Another study conducted in 1993 in Atlanta found that 29% of female sex workers were HIV positive. A study conducted by John R. Talbott showed a close correspondence between the percent of women who are engaged in sex work and the percent of the female population that is HIV infected. Regions of the world with the greatest percentage of women involved in commercial sex work are the same regions with the highest rates of HIV/AIDS among sex workers. For example, Africa has the greatest number of commercial sex workers in the female population and the greatest prevalence of HIV/AIDS among women, whereas the United States and Western Europe have the least number of commercial sex workers and among the lowest rates of HIV/AIDS in women. Research has now shown that insufficient food is a driving force in women engaging commercial sex work and subsequent HIV infection. The association between commercial sex work and AIDS completely contradicts Duesberg's statements that there is no AIDS problem among prostitutes.

Common in denialism, Duesberg's arguments for how AIDS develops often contain partially truthful elements. Some partial truths in the Duesbergian view of AIDS are reflected in the facts, including:

- **Duesberg**: A retrovirus would cause rapid disease, not a slow progressing disease. **Fact**: HIV does cause disease throughout its course, but there is a long clinical latency period during which the person with HIV remains clinically healthy because the immune system is not yet disabled, although continuously damaged.
- **Duesberg**: Exposure to toxins and drugs including antiretroviral medications can suppress the immune system and cause AIDS. **Fact**: Illicit drugs and toxins can suppress the immune system and can facilitate HIV disease, but they do not cause loss of CD4/T-Helper cells like that seen in AIDS. Drugs used to treat HIV, especially in the early years of AIDS had serious side effects, but they do not cause the loss of CD4/T-Helper cells.

The extremism that characterizes denialism that is typified by Duesberg obscures the truth and complexity of how HIV causes AIDS.

The Grant that Never Was

In 1993, Duesberg did submit a grant application to study AIDS to the National Institute on Drug Abuse (NIDA), one of the National Institutes of Health. What Duesberg proposed was a study to test his recreational drugs theory of AIDS. Though the grant application was definitively rejected by the institute, it is important to understand just how and why the institute turned it down. Some denialists have claimed that the rejection amounts to proof of a government conspiracy to silence Duesberg. For example, consider how the whole complicated affair is described by the distinguished Yale University mathematician Serge Lang, a friend of Duesberg who spent extended periods of time in the math department at UC Berkeley, who informally but reasonably enough provides this brief description of what was being proposed:

> The purpose of the application was to examine the effect of some drugs (nitrites) on some animals, to see if they cause AIDS-related diseases involving both immunodeficiency, and cancer type diseases. As Duesberg once said, 'we'll feed poppers to mice.'[14]

The research set out in this grant proposal would test Duesberg's ideas on what causes AIDS. The history of Duesberg's grant applications can be found in the archives of the UC Berkeley Library. Lang's narrative of the scientific review of the grant application leads to the conclusion that peer reviewers were unfair in their treatment of the application and its investigator. Duesberg himself tells us that his grant had been encouraged by NIDA and endorsed by leading scientists, including the Editor of the journal *Science*. According to Lang, the rigorous grant-review process noted the importance of the proposed research, stating that "the major strength of this proposal is that it addresses the important public health problems of whether nitrite abuse acts as a cofactor in AIDS pathogenesis." Lang generally mischaracterizes the entire grant review, however, stating "Thus the proposal did not even receive a 'priority score,' or a full review, but was summarily rejected at the initial stage." In fact, the grant was fully reviewed. The review led to the decision not to render a score for the grant, the fate of half of all grants submitted to the NIH. All grants that do not receive a score are not discussed further by the grant review committee. Nevertheless, the grant was fully reviewed. Ultimately, the grant did not pass the peer-review process and was not funded. The question is, Why?

One concern that the NIDA grant reviewers expressed was that the basis for the proposed research was biased, presenting a "one-sided rationale" for the research. The reviewers stated that "A more thorough and balanced description of the pertinent literature would instill more confidence in the rationale and design of the proposed studies." Lang objected to this concern, stating "It was not Duesberg's responsibility to present a many-sided rationale for doing the proposed experiment." Lang's objection is, however, invalid. It is incumbent on grant applicants to articulate a clear and compelling rationale for the proposed research while impartially presenting the known body of research. The contributions of new research can only be considered in the context of an unbiased account of existing knowledge.

Another major concern expressed by the grant reviewers was that Duesberg and his co-researchers had not carried out preliminary studies leading to their proposed research project. Lang also found this criticism outrageous, stating:

> One objection was that "the proposal does not describe any preliminary studies," although the Summary Statement recognized that "the preliminary studies section describes experiments performed by other groups that should be in the background and significance section." Indeed, the proposal described systematically many preliminary studies by other groups. Why it should be a cause for rejection that Duesberg's lab did not do preliminary studies when others have done them is beyond me, and I regard this reason as illegitimate. It is now for the community of scientists to evaluate the legitimacy of this reason.[15]

Contrary to Lang's interpretation, the Preliminary Studies section of a grant application is critical to demonstrating the capacity of the researchers who are applying for the grant to complete the proposed work as well as an evaluation of the proposed research methods. The NIH grant application instructions clearly describe the importance of preliminary studies conducted by the investigators for the proposed research. Grant reviewers attend carefully to the pilot research, or preliminary studies, conducted by the researchers because these studies tell reviewers whether the research lab submitting the application has the capacity to do the science.[16] In this case, including this information in the Preliminary Studies section of the grant would be particularly important because Duesberg is not a toxicologist or immunologist, the specializations that would be most well equipped to perform studies of drugs and the immune system.

In addition, Lang noted that the grant reviewers claimed that "the proposed design of the mouse experiments is not clear." The reviewers were concerned about the order of experimental manipulations and the implication of the order for interpreting the results. Lang stated "Just because there are several variations which could give rise to several types of experiments is not a justification to prevent one among many possible experiments from being carried out." However, Lang seems to have missed the point. The reviewers expressed concern about whether the proposed experiments would yield interpretable findings, not merely the choice among many experiments.

Duesberg revised his grant application and resubmitted it in 1994, but again it was turned down. The reason was simple: Revised grant applications that are not responsive to the first-round comments are extremely unlikely to move forward. The reviewers were very clear that Duesberg would need to do preliminary studies to demonstrate the promise of his ideas, a requirement of all grants like the type he applied for. Specifically stating "I think the investigators could perform these tests if they did some preliminary studies and if they first answered the criticisms in a future revised application." There is no evidence that Duesberg ever conducted the necessary preliminary studies and was therefore unresponsive to the initial reviews.

Still another reason for rejection of the proposal was that it was not breaking new ground. The novelty of Duesberg's proposed research is questionable. In 1993, NIDA was already funding a study on inhalable nitrites and their effects on immune function; it showed that nitrite inhalants did not demonstrate an immune suppressive response like that seen in AIDS. NIDA was also funding a study titled "Immunotoxicity of Abused Nitrite Inhalants," awarded to Lee Soderberg of the University of Arkansas Medical School. Duesberg's AIDS grant was not seen as innovative or cutting-edge in the highly competitive world of NIDA-funded research.[17]

It is therefore apparent that understanding why Duesberg's proposal did not receive funding does not require a broad government conspiracy.

Character Flaw?

It is not that Duesberg is entirely wrong on AIDS. Rather, he is marginalized by the extremity and exclusivity of his views, and the disrespect for science he shows in promoting them at the expense of other, more significant and compelling, explanations. Duesberg is alone, among scientists trained in virology, in claiming that HIV does not have a role in causing AIDS (and alone among cancer researchers in claiming that Aneuploidy is the sole cause of cancer). What explains his tendency to take such extreme and exclusivist views, which opposes the mainstream? Why does he take on and then dismiss essentially the entire scientific community?

Before he even questioned HIV as the cause of AIDS, Duesberg was highly skeptical. Celia Farber has noted that Duesberg is following in a German tradition. Like Gunther Stent and Max Delbruck, two world renowned biologists who immigrated from Germany to the U.S. She also pointed out that Duesberg has a tendency to stake a line in the sand and challenge anyone who dares to cross it. He values – one might even say he thrives on – vigorous dissidence and vigorous debate. But while he is intellectually vibrant, he is also entrenched in his own thoughts.

In a recent *Discover* Magazine article about Duesberg, Robert Weinberg of the Whitehead Institute calls him a contrarian with a corrosive and acidic wit. Contrarian may be an understatement. You almost get the feeling that if suddenly it were discovered that AIDS is caused by toxic drugs Duesberg would refute the evidence and pose an alternative theory.

Duesberg pursued the idea that retroviruses cause cancer only until the idea became mainstream. At his Aneuploidy conference in Oakland, Duesberg was the first to ask questions of every speaker, sometimes even before they finished speaking. There was an eagerness or even impulsiveness to his challenging their presentations. There were even times when his assistant took the microphone to give others a chance to speak. The intense curiosity that seemed to drive Duesberg's probing pushed people to think deeper than they would have otherwise. What easily could have been a dry academic discussion, Duesberg turned into a raucous intellectual sporting event.

Is it possible that Peter Duesberg himself does not seriously question whether HIV causes AIDS? In a position paper that he wrote for a South African meeting, he referred to the classic novel *The Plague* by Albert Camus as the most readable modern depiction of an epidemic. Addressing a country where hundreds of people die of AIDS each day, Duesberg's reference to a work of fiction seems quite telling.[18] Was he signaling that we should not take him too seriously? Perhaps he pushes on his academic rivals only because he enjoys the argument – as a kind of sport, debate for the sake of debate. Observing his exchanges with colleagues over such matters as the role of Aneuploidy in cancer reveals that he takes a certain joy in scholarly debate. He dominates the dialogue and challenges all other positions in defending his own. Intellectually, to me, at least, Duesberg is like a big-game fisherman who loves the fight but ultimately loses the battle because he will not give any slack. But to leave matters there, to see him as what used to be called "a character," is to be too charitable. The word "character" has other meanings.

Duesberg also demonstrates utter disregard for science in his selective manipulation of research findings. In AIDS research, there are several examples of Duesberg taking a single sentence out of context or using a single result from a study to suggest that he is right about AIDS. For example, in his 2008 interview with *Discover* Magazine, Duesberg stated that Kaposi's sarcoma, a form of cancer found in men with AIDS, is caused by drug abuse and the declines in this disease parallel the decline in some drugs used by gay men. However, it is conclusively established that Kaposi's sarcoma is caused by a type of sexually transmitted herpes virus and its decline parallels increases in safer sex among gay men. Similarly, he misuses sound research findings that indicate changes in the amount of virus in the blood following initiation of HIV treatment do not predict living longer in people with HIV/AIDS. Or when Duesberg discussed in a 2007 interview research published in the *Journal of the American Medical Association* that found HIV concentrations in blood, or viral load, to have no correlation with developing AIDS. Duesberg claims the study shows there is no HIV in relation to AIDS whereas the researchers refute this misinterpretation and state the opposite – HIV causes AIDS but in a way too complex to be indexed by viral load alone.

Duesberg also claimed in his 2006 Lew Rockwell conference presentation that this same research finding refutes the effectiveness of HIV treatments, whereas the results actually show just the opposite when we account for increasing numbers of people dying from lethal tuberculosis. Surely he understands scientific findings reported in medical journals, and this leads me to only one conclusion that he intentionally misrepresents science for his own personal gain, or more likely aggrandizement. This is the behavior that raises questions about Duesberg's character in the other sense of the word. Duesberg needs to be right and he loves the debate, even at the cost of losing rationality and ultimately at the cost of doing great harm.

Duesberg the Victim

Much of Duesberg's support comes from defenders of open expression and academic freedom. Duesberg's own account of his downward-spiraling career points to a plot against him for merely questioning HIV as the cause of AIDS. Having failed to receive grant support from the NIH – years after he simultaneously abandoned researching genetic causes of cancer, Duesberg turned toward Aneuploidy as the cause of cancer and declared that HIV cannot cause AIDS. He holds that it is not his ideas and theories that are the source of his failure, but that he himself is the target of a conspiracy spearheaded by the scientific orthodoxy. Celia Farber's description of his experience with the final NIH grant review in 1993 takes up the theme of Duesberg as victim of the U.S. government:

> The Outstanding Investigator Grant Duesberg had received was designed to allow elite scientists to focus on their work with the cushion of a seven year grant, the idea being that they shouldn't spend precious time on grant-seeking. So the NIH was unable, legally, to close the spigot of funds to Duesberg until 1993. But when Duesberg's grant came up for renewal, he had the proverbial "snowball's chance in summer," as Bialy put it. The review committee included one AIDS researcher who had financial ties to the company that made AZT, a drug Duesberg continually criticized for its extreme toxicity, and one who had mothered a child by the scientist who spawned the HIV–AIDS hypothesis, Robert Gallo. Three reviewers never even read the proposal. Duesberg was doomed. The US government unceremoniously pulled the plug and would never again give him a single research dollar. He went from being among the government's most highly funded scientists to being completely cut off. A kind of anti-Duesbergism swept the field and grew to a near-frenzy.[19]

Duesberg claims that all reviewers of government grants have an inherent conflict of interest. Peer reviewers, he says, must protect their own ideas and research interests, and therefore criticize grant proposals that challenge the status quo. Duesberg states that grant-review committees are hand-picked, or "deputized," by the government to bias the direction of science. The goal of peer review, according to Duesberg, is to squelch new ideas and limit innovative thinking in science. Speaking from experience, I have to add that no one enjoys having an NIH research grant go unfunded. Nevertheless, a government conspiracy against any researcher, even Duesberg, is hard to imagine. Grant-review committees consist of several established researchers, and there is no contingency between serving on grant review committees and receiving grants. Some of the most prominent and well-funded researchers I know have never served on grant review committees. At least three designated expert reviewers write detailed comments and critiques. The reviewers discuss each grant that is found meritorious openly in front of a full committee of peer scientists as well as outside observers. While the process does protect the identity of reviewers to assure their candid critique, the reviewers openly discuss the grants with each other.

Duesberg is therefore pointing to a conspiracy of 30,000 NIH peer reviewers who serve on such committees each year to review over 80,000 grants. Grant-review committees also change annually, with no one member allowed to serve more than a few years. Also, contrary to what Duesberg and his followers say, creativity is not only encouraged in NIH grants, innovation is one of the required review criteria for merit. An orchestrated effort to keep one scientist unfunded would indeed require a widespread conspiracy involving the U.S. government and a very large segment of the entire scientific enterprise.

Nevertheless, Duesberg and his inner-circle maintain that there is a conspiracy against him and anyone else who questions that HIV causes AIDS. For example, David Rasnick, Duesberg's long time associate who has become involved in his own brand of AIDS pseudoscience, has said:

> The AIDS blunder shows that we need to rethink and restructure our institutions of government, science, health, academe, journalism and media. We must replace the National Institutes of Health as the primary gatekeeper of research funding with numerous competing sources of funding. We must restructure the peer review processes of scientific publishing and funding so that they do not promote and protect any particular dogma or fashion of thought or exclude competing ideas.[20]

Another close colleague and biographer of Duesberg, Harvey Bialy, views peer review as a corrupt and conspiring entity. For example, in 2006 he stated in an article posted at the Lew Rockwell social libertarian web site:

> Today's scientists are almost wholly dependent upon the goodwill of government researchers and powerful peer-review boards, who control a financial network binding together the National Institutes of Health, academia, and the biotech and pharmaceutical industries. Many scientists live in fear of losing their funding.[21]

Duesberg has himself described the peer review process and the basis for a conspiracy against him:

> The peer review system derives its power from the little known practice of governments to deputize their authority to distribute funds for research to committees of "experts." These experts are academic researchers distinguished by outstanding contributions to the current establishment. They alone review the merits of research applications from their peers, and they have the right to elect each other to review committees. Outwardly, this "peer review system" appears to the unsuspecting government and taxpayer as the equivalent of a jury system – free of all conflicts of interest. But, in view of the many professional and commercial investments in and benefits from their expertise, and even of the rewards from their universities and institutions for the corresponding overheads and partnerships – all legal in the US since president Reagan – "peer reviewers" do not fund applications that challenge their own interests. Since "peer review" is protected by anonymity, does not allow the applicant personal representation or an independent representative, nor a say or even a veto in the selection of the "jury," and does not allow an appeal, its powers to defend the orthodoxy are unlimited. The corporate equivalent of academia's "peer review system" would be to give General Motors and Ford the authority to review and veto all innovations by less established carmakers competing for the consumer.[22]

A victim of a peer-review conspiracy, Duesberg has proposed an alternative to the system. In an interview with Joseph Mercola in 2001, he offered the following procedure to replace peer review in science:

> The ONLY solution would be to free scientific spending from vested interests (i.e., the "expert" peer review). Science would have to be judged by "expert citizens" (i.e., those who can earn taxes (sic), read and write and have common sense, just as those who serve because they are non-experts, i.e., us, the people in the legal jury system). NOT by those who have exceedingly large vested interests, like their professional egos, their grants, their summer salaries, their companies, their patents, their "frequent flier" benefits, and their awards on their minds.[23]

Almost needless to say, it is unlikely in the extreme that scientists will ever agree to have the merit of future research funded by taxpayer dollars determined by expert citizens. I do not even know a single taxpayer who would want to see that happen.

A Groundswell of Support

Denialism took root in the late 1980s and early 1990s. Without any research to support their claims, Duesberg and his inner circle formed The Group for the Scientific Reappraisal of the HIV/AIDS Hypothesis. The Group, as it is now called, has been active in letter-writing, law suits, and Internet postings, but has not done research on AIDS. How then does The Group influence public opinion and attract attention? The major thrust of denialist activity comes in the form of journalism. Dissent, betrayal, conspiracy, suppression of ideas – all make for a good story. Invariably, Duesberg is portrayed as a mild-mannered victim of a conspiracy that wants to keep the truth about AIDS from us. Interpersonally, Duesberg is very engaging and charming. It is very easy to like being around this guy. And there is an element of adventure in denialism, with a world painted in strokes of good and evil. Major magazines such as *Spin, Harpers* and *Discover,* and newspapers such as *The London Sunday Times* print denialist accounts of AIDS and lend an air of credibility to their pleas for freedom of expression. Who, after all, wants to come out in favor of suppression? However, there is also the matter of journalistic responsibility that needs to be considered, the responsibility for verifying facts and avoiding stories that bring to readers nothing more than sensational accusations. Journalism has helped to fuel support for denialist claims by reporting conspiracy theories and unsupported theories about AIDS as if they were credible and backed up by science.

Peter Duesberg, with his credentials, his charm, and his very real accomplishments, became a convenient public figure providing scientific cover for prominent denialists in the popular press. Most notably Christine Maggiore assimilated Peter Duesberg's views for her own tragic story, ultimately leading others to deny that HIV causes AIDS and that being HIV positive is of no consequence. Duesberg explains how Maggiore tested HIV positive and remained healthy. He does not explain how Maggiore's child died at the age of three from what the Los Angeles Coroner determined was AIDS.

Duesberg's ideas have also intersected with political and religious conservatism. Followers of intelligent design, the new creationism, gravitate to Duesberg because he implicates man's own behaviors in causing AIDS and cancer. It is impure lifestyles and harm to the environment, then, rather than the chance flukes of nature, such as mutated genes and viruses, that have visited these terrible diseases on us. Duesberg offers biblical allusions in describing Aneuploidy as the cause rather than the consequence of cancer. For example, he stated "carcinogenesis is like Genesis: a cancer cell would be generated from a normal cell by karyotype (chromosomal) alterations, much like a new phylogenic species."[24] Denialists have emerged on highly charged conservative web sites, such as Rebecca Culshaw's debut on the Lew Rockwell web site. Tom Bethell, a conservative journalist, has written several pieces that directly support Peter Duesberg, providing a bridge for Peter Duesberg from the obscure world of denialism and Aneuploidy to religious right wing conservatism. Duesberg's views that AIDS and cancer are caused by lifestyles and toxins also appeal to environmental extremists such as David Crowe who suggest that it is better to live and die with cancer than take "toxic cell-killing chemicals" in chemotherapy.

It is also noteworthy that much of the groundswell of support for Duesberg has come from his German colleagues, suggesting a nationalistic source for at least some of his support. As a German-born and German-trained scientist whose father served in the German Army during WW-II, Duesberg may evoke a sort of nationalist sentimental loyalty among some fellow country-men. Moreover, the fact that Aneuploidy was originally discussed in Germany in the 1800s and early 1900s may evoke a certain sense of pride. The number of German colleagues who rally around Duesberg is notable: vitamin sales entrepreneur Matthias Rath; virologist Stefan Lanka; Heinrich Kremer medical director of the Federal Clinics for Juvenile and Young Adult Drug Offenders for five German counties; Charles Geshekter, professor of African history at the California State University, Chico; University of Miami professor Rudolf Werner, trained in biochemistry at the University of Freiburg; Heinz Ludwig Sänger, Emeritus Professor of Molecular Biology and Virology and a former director of the Department of Viroid Research at the Max-Planck-Institutes for Biochemy near Munich; Henry Bauer, Austrian born academic; and Claus Koehnlein, Department of Oncology at the University of Kiel. It is not surprising that Duesberg would know many Germans given that he spends his summers in Germany. What is surprising is the number of credentialed professionals who support his fringe ideas on AIDS and cancer.

Another group of Duesberg supporters can be traced back to colleagues at UC Berkeley. This group includes his longtime associate David Rasnick, who also worked with German vitamin salesman Matthias Rath in South Africa. Rasnick has in fact spent time at Berkeley; but he has also claimed to be a visiting scholar in the Department of Molecular and Cell Biology, and this is disputed by the university. Another previously mentioned supporter, Harvey Bialy, received his degree in molecular biology from Berkeley in 1970. The famed Yale mathematician Serge Lang spent time in the math department at UC Berkeley where he came to know Duesberg. Then there is Berkeley Law Professor Phillip Johnson, who became a born-again Christian and a supporter of Intelligent Design, he wrote articles about HIV/AIDS dissent and government cover-ups in direct support of Duesberg. Seth Roberts is a Psychology Professor at Berkeley and he has made contributions to denialism. Also a supporter is Andrew J. Maniotis, who graduated from Berkeley in 1991 and is a vocal denialist who sits on the Advisory Board of Christine Maggiore's Alive and Well organization.

Has Duesberg Been Given His Due?

Peter Duesberg's chief gripe, and the source of much of his support, is that scientists have simply not taken him seriously. This is undeniably true. But should we wonder why, when a respected scientist makes the claim that HIV does not cause AIDS, no one listens? Duesberg has repeatedly called for a public debate on the cause of AIDS. Celia Farber has even suggested an Internet-based debate, where Duesberg could go at it with blog-like postings – point-counter-point style in a public forum.

However, a public debate on whether HIV causes AIDS by a respectable AIDS scientist and Duesberg will likely never happen. For one reason, AIDS scientists do not see Duesberg as credible. Second, AIDS scientists simply do not see anything to debate about when it comes to HIV causing AIDS. There are no science-based disputes. There are no contradictory data. There are no opposing studies. There is just Duesberg and a few others who theorize that HIV does not cause AIDS. In order to have a meaningful discussion of a disagreement, you have to start with some crucial points on which you do agree, and these are lacking.

Time taken away from AIDS research to debate Duesberg seems unjustifiable. He does not have major research grants and he has a small lab funded by a private donor with two lab assistants and no students. Most others who cry out for a debate on HIV causing AIDS have similar situations – unfunded labs, emeritus faculty positions, self-employment, freelance journalism, and oftentimes retirement. Perhaps the main reason why a debate on HIV causing AIDS simply will not happen is that the debate itself would give unwarranted credence to the very question of whether HIV causes AIDS. The sad and destructive consequence of South Africa's former President Mbeki orchestrating an AIDS debate in his own AIDS Advisory Panel is that it created a façade of legitimacy for denialists and pseudoscientists.

Still, over the years, Peter Duesberg has been answered on all of his key points. There have been numerous responses from the scientific community aimed at settling the question by directly responding to Duesberg's arguments. For example, in 1994 the National Institutes of Health created a document titled *The Evidence that HIV Causes AIDS* that responds directly to Duesberg and the information is regularly updated. The most thorough and compelling examination of Duesberg's claims was conducted in the late 1990s for the journal *Science*, which undertook an extensive investigation that involved over 50 experts who evaluated the evidence for what causes AIDS and corresponded directly with Duesberg throughout the process. Perhaps the most credible science journalist of his time, Jon Cohen, asked Duesberg for an interview and Duesberg accepted. Cohen provided questions ahead of time in writing to which Duesberg responded in writing and interviews. Cohen submitted 10 single-space pages of questions that Duesberg answered in 11 single-spaced pages. Then Cohen submitted a second batch of questions that Duesberg answered. Jon Cohen told Peter Duesberg that he would take him seriously on every point he was making.[25] Examining several lines of evidence, Cohen concluded that refusing to accept that HIV causes

AIDS in the face of the entire scientific community has made Duesberg a cult hero to those who oppose big government, big pharma, and medical science.

In 1996, Stephen O'Brien and James Goedert published an article in the journal *Current Opinion in Immunology* that extensively examined the evidence at the time that HIV causes AIDS and proclaimed that the important Koch's Postulates were indeed fulfilled.[26] O'Brien and Goedert laid out the evidence that shows that almost all AIDS patients have HIV antibodies and those with HIV antibodies have confirmed HIV infection. In fact, there are only 16 known cases of AIDS in which people have not developed HIV antibodies, although they do have the virus.[27] Although HIV is not the only cause of immune suppression, HIV definitely causes the specific type of immune suppression that causes AIDS – depleted CD4/T-Helper cells. HIV has been isolated from AIDS patients. Transmission of the virus is also now proven through accidental exposure. For example, in the early 1990s over 1000 children under age 13 received HIV contaminated blood or other medical exposures to HIV in Romania. These children developed AIDS, whereas children not exposed to contaminated blood did not develop AIDS.

Peter Duesberg's scientific credentials, especially his Full Professorship at a respected institution and membership in the National Academy of Sciences, are surely factors in the number of credible responses he has received to his off-beat claims. There is no scientific evidence available to counter the thousands of studies that have shown HIV causes AIDS. There is also no research to support the idea that drug use or malnutrition cause AIDS-specific damage to the immune system. Duesberg is not the first scientist to question a prevailing view of a disease and we can thankfully trust that there will always be dissident scientists. But we are also fortunate that few other dissidents will waste precious time and divert limited resources to chase after answered questions in a self-indulging quest for debate.

Peter Duesberg's legacies will be that he both discovered the first cancer causing gene and that he brought a sort of legitimacy to a band of sad denialists and wacky pseudoscientists. How one man could be the source of so many lives saved and so many lives lost is the greatest paradox and human tragedy in this whole contorted affair.

AIDS Pseudoscience

3

Only two things are infinite, the universe and human stupidity, and
I'm not sure about the former.
Albert Einstein

What is science? What is not science? Who gets to decide? Defining science is an undertaking far beyond the scope of this book. Fortunately, we do not have to define science to understand pseudoscience. Simply put, pseudoscience – also known as fringe science or alternative science – masquerades as real science but because of its defects it is not science at all. The most important of these defects is its lack of thoughtful experimentation, the very foundation of science. Michael Shermer, noted author and skeptic of the extravagant claims of pseudoscience, defines it as claims that appear scientific even though they lack supporting evidence and plausibility. Pseudoscience does not advance, it does not move forward; there is no accumulation of knowledge. Pseudoscientific thinking relies instead on anecdotes, scientific-sounding language, bold statements without supporting evidence, and after the fact reasoning.

Pseudoscience, which is not science at all, differs from bad science and junk science, which are science but utilize faulty methodologies to draw incorrect conclusions. Summarized by Shermer and others, the many different fields of pseudoscience, so to speak, share common characteristics:

- The goals of pseudoscience are most likely ideological, cultural, or commercial.
- A pseudoscience evolves very little since first established. Small amounts of flawed research and experimentation are generally performed to justify existing beliefs.
- Within a pseudoscience, challenges to accepted dogma are considered hostile acts if not heresy, and always lead to bitter disputes.

- The major tenets and principles of the field are often not falsifiable and are unlikely to ever be shown wrong.
- Individual egos and personalities tend to shape pseudoscientific concepts.
- Individuals who are not in contact with mainstream science propagate pseudoscience.
- Pseudoscience invokes authority (a famous name, for example) for support.
- Pseudoscientific explanations tend to be vague and ambiguous, often using scientific terms in dubious contexts.
- Pseudoscience uses vague, exaggerated or un-testable claims that lack precise measurements.
- A pseudoscience uses selective experimental findings that seem to support its own claims while suppressing or refusing to consider contradictory data.

Pseudoscience is usually associated with reports of extraordinary unprovable events. Sightings of UFOs, alien abductions, astrology, psychic predictions, paranormal activity, and monster sightings all come to mind. Outlandish claims about the cause and cure of diseases constitute another domain of pseudoscience.

Pseudoscience flat-out denies an entire body of accepted facts, drawing it in close kinship to denialism. Like denialism, pseudoscience evades, ignores, and avoids undeniable facts. Quite different from denialism, pseudoscience requires that the person making claims have at least the appearance of scientific credentials. Denialist journalists who report AIDS pseudoscience are accomplices but they are not pseudoscientists. Pseudoscience involves picking and choosing research findings to support beliefs in the absence of original research. As Peter Duesberg's close associate David Rasnick said at his recent cancer and Aneuploidy conference, he relies on the research of others because he does not do research himself. The selective use and misuse of science ultimately forms the basis for concocting pseudoscience.

Conducting Research Versus Concocting Pseudoscience

To the casual reader, AIDS pseudoscience is becoming increasingly more difficult to distinguish from AIDS science. In science, editors rely on peer review to determine the quality and contribution of a particular piece of research. Pseudoscientists have exploited scientific outlets by publishing their views as letters to the editor of some of the most prestigious journals in science. Pseudoscience creeps into the scientific literature through commentaries, correspondences, and in other open, non-peer reviewed forums. In the late 1990s, editors of scientific journals limited, or in some cases eliminated, the publication of unfounded claims about the cause of AIDS. One example comes from the *South African Medical Journal* (*SAMJ*), where the Editor wrote:

> Medical journals have a responsibility to put all sides of important questions to readers. However, there comes a time when continuing to pander to tangential viewpoints serves no useful purpose and may indeed be harmful. At an early stage of the propagation of the beliefs of the AIDS dissidents it could be argued that those supporting establishment views should be informed of the dissidents' beliefs in order to test their hypotheses, or blow them out of the water. That stage was reached some time ago when the small group of dissidents had spent their tolerance capital for space in mainstream medical journals. With the medical and scientific facts so clearly demonstrated, printing their repetitive arguments detracts from the main task of dealing with the pandemic. It also takes time and effort repeatedly to have to refute outlandish claims. The *SAMJ [South African Medical Journal]* therefore does not accept such material.[1]

Pseudoscientists seek publication outlets that circumvent scientific peer review. Books are one such outlet that is not contingent on peer review. Others include web sites, magazines, and self-produced documents such as brochures, newsletters, and monographs – all familiar homes for pseudoscience. Worst of all, there are scientific peer reviewed journals that do not subject all work to peer-review, reserving space for articles to publish at the Editor's discretion. AIDS pseudoscientists have successfully exploited all of these avenues of publication to create a self-perpetuating corpus of confusion.

It is worth taking time to examine an instance of how this corpus of bogus scholarship is repackaged in a publication, and which in turn is itself added to the corpus. Rebecca Culshaw's 2007 book *Science Sold Out: Does HIV Really Cause AIDS?* is published by a New Age publisher, Atlantic Books based in Berkeley California, of course. Culshaw, a college math teacher, summarizes denialist claims dating back to the 1980s without offering any new ideas or evidence. Among her 100 sources in her reference list, 41 were published by recognized AIDS denialists, 22 were from scientifically accepted works published in the 1980s and only 10 sources reference scientific articles from 2000 forward. In another 2007 book, *The Origin, Persistence, and Failings of HIV/AIDS Theory*, Henry Bauer similarly ignores science. His book claims to prove HIV cannot cause AIDS and relies on 436 sources, of which two out of three predate the year 2000. Only 38 of his sources, that is about 9%, are from scientific journals published since 2000. Bauer's book appears science-based and claims to be scientific, but it violates every basic rule of science, statistics, and logical thinking! Bauer misuses selective rates of HIV testing to draw conclusions about AIDS diagnoses from completely different populations. AIDS pseudoscientific books help create a façade of credibility for denialism.

Of course, following the rules of scientific publication does not absolutely guarantee that scientific papers are of high quality. There are plenty of instances where peer review fails, such as when reviewers hold undisclosed conflicts of interest or fail to attend to the nuances and details of a particular research study. Every scientific journal editor surely has stories about papers that, in hindsight, probably should not have made it through peer-review. The same can likely be said for research grants. But there is something fundamentally wrong with scholarship that avoids peer review. Why rely on back alley outlets if what you have to say will advance the field? As discussed in Chapter 4, AIDS pseudoscientists are quick to point out that their work is suppressed by a conspiracy to censor the truth about AIDS. Needless to say there is no evidence, other than the rejected work of pseudoscientists, that any such censorship has occurred. The peer review system is far from perfect, but no one has come up with any better way to improve the quality of advancing science. In that sense, the static world of pseudoscience is served well by outlets that do not subject their work to peer-review. I have divided AIDS pseudoscience into "fields" that mirror the fields of science that are mimicked, namely virology, immunology, pharmacology, and epidemiology.

Pseudo-virology: HIV Does Not Exist

Virology is the scientific discipline that is concerned with the study of viruses and how they cause disease. I therefore include those pseudoscientists who make claims about the virus as pseudo-virologists. Few AIDS pseudoscientists actually deny that HIV exists. Even Peter Duesberg, for all of his odd ideas, recognizes that the virus exists. Nonetheless, there are a few who do doubt the very existence of HIV. Although there are confusing inconsistencies in their writings, the so-called Perth Group most consistently denies the very existence of the virus. The esoteric Australian academics that make up the Perth Group includes its three founding members, biophysicist Eleni Papadopulos-Eleopulos, emergency physician Valendar Turner, and Professor of Pathology John Papadimitriou. They tell a convoluted tale using various rhetorical techniques to sound scientific regarding the first studies that reported isolating HIV. Turner, for example, concluded that there were flaws in Robert Gallo's initial research on HIV and that the evidence claiming HIV exists is inconclusive:

Even if the Gallo team had proved the existence of a new retrovirus, on what basis did they claim it was the cause of AIDS? Even if virus had been isolated from all patients and all patients had antibodies, which they didn't because in the fourth paper, the data showed only 88% of AIDS patients had antibodies (and on a single ELISA test which no one now regards as specific), is this sufficient proof that HIV causes AIDS? If the bank manager and his constant, faithful offsider are present at the bank robbery, is this proof that the manager robbed the bank?[2]

The Perth Group had gone so far as to offer a $20,000 prize to anyone who can prove that HIV does exist, challenging:

> So confident am I that no such electron-micrograph evidence for the existence of 'HIV' can be produced by adhering strictly to the Etienne de Harven methodology, I am prepared to offer the sum of £10,000 to the first person to submit just such a micrograph, prepared under stringent laboratory conditions. I do not want 'markers' for 'viral activity' which are at very best, inaccurate. I want visual evidence of myriad active, infectious viral particles, clearly morphologically defined recovered from a fresh sample of bodily fluid, unadulterated with any other kinds of cells.[3]

Humorously, Duesberg challenged the Perth Group that HIV actually has been isolated and proven to exist, but of course he believes it does not cause AIDS. But the Perth Group rebuked Duesberg and denied him the cash prize.

Heinz Ludwig Sänger, Professor of Molecular Biology and Virology formerly at the Max-Planck-Institutes for Biochemy near München Germany similarly concluded that the past 20 years of HIV/AIDS research has shown that the existence of HIV has not been proven "without doubt," and that it cannot be responsible for the immunodeficiency that characterizes AIDS. Roberto Giraldo, vitamin pusher and pseudoscientist, at least at times states that HIV does not exist and has recommended to doctors:

> It is absolutely necessary to convince the patient and the community that they are not infected with 'the virus that causes AIDS.' The feeling of being infected with the virus that supposedly causes AIDS, in addition to being an immunological stressor, blocks participation of brain and mind in the healing process. The 'HIV/AIDS hysteria' must be stopped immediately.[4]

Giraldo, like the Perth Group, claims that the answer to AIDS is to stop the oxidizing processes of stress and drugs – especially the drugs used to treat HIV and instead to use detoxifying antioxidants as well as non-toxic remedies. What non-toxic remedies does Giraldo push? His long list includes acupuncture, digitopunture, Chinese traditional medicine, herbal medicine, Indian ayurvedic medicine, hyperthermia, oxygen therapy, massage therapy, homeopathy, naturopathic and colon therapy, music therapy, color therapy, gem therapy, aromatherapy, hypnosis therapy, light therapy, yoga, magnetic field therapy, orthomolecular medicine, cell therapy, and spiritual care.

The conclusion that HIV does not exist leads to the dangerous and equally illogical question as to why should a person get tested for HIV at all? Crying out for an end to HIV testing is the steam-head of denialism that is most obviously fueled by pseudo-immunology.

Pseudo-immunology I: HIV Exists but HIV Tests Are Invalid

Immunology is the branch of biomedical sciences that is concerned with all aspects of the immune system and its defenses against disease, including the production of antibodies. Thus, AIDS pseudoscientists who claim that "a person can test positive for HIV antibodies, but that does not mean that he or she has an HIV infection" have delved into the world of pseudo-immunology. Claiming that having HIV antibodies does not necessarily mean that a person has an infection is aimed at discouraging people from taking the HIV test and it encourages people who have tested HIV positive to disregard their diagnosis. AIDS pseudoscientists use a confusing mosaic of scientific sounding statements taken out of context to portray HIV antibody tests as unreliable. HIV testing involves at least two stages, which when done properly are among the most reliable diagnostic tests in medicine. The chance for an HIV negative person testing HIV positive on a correctly performed test (showing what is called a false positive result) is less than a hundredth of a percent. That means that HIV antibody tests are 99.99% accurate![5]

If the HIV test is so accurate, how do AIDS pseudoscientists dare say that the test is grossly inaccurate? The most common argument that pseudoscientists use to discredit HIV testing is to claim that the tests are circular in their reasoning. The Perth Group, for example, states that AIDS patients surely test positive for HIV antibodies but that does not mean that they have HIV infection. They exploit the differences between individually licensed HIV test kits to falsely claim that there are no standards for determining a positive test result. Their argument is that people with AIDS surely have a plethora of antibodies because they have so many different infections, so the HIV test is confusing other diseases with HIV. To someone who does not understand HIV testing this may sound concerning, but is actually nonsense.

The Perth Group, Harvey Bialy, Rebecca Culshaw, Henry Bauer and others rely on research conducted in 1985 and 1986 to show that people can receive a positive HIV test when they are in fact HIV negative. Cross-reactions occur when the test confuses the wrong antibody for the ones that the test is designed for. Cross-reactions with the HIV antibody tests were more common in the early 1980s when the tests were new. AIDS pseudoscientists use the most bizarre examples of cross-reaction to distract attention away from the actual accuracy of the tests. Two common examples of immunologic cross-reactions that they use are indeed bizarre. For one, they state that HIV testing for antbodies is undermined because antibodies to an ox heart extract (cardiolipin) predicts the development of syphilis, but of course the extract has nothing to do with syphilis. A second strange example of cross-reaction they use is that patients with infectious mononucleosis develop antibodies that cross-react with sheep and horse red blood cells. The point they are making is that antibody tests can produce false positive results when the antibodies cross-react with antibodies to some other antigen. Cross-reaction can and does happen with the HIV antibody test, such as when a person is tested for HIV soon after receiving any one of a number of vaccinations. In these very rare instances, the HIV test can mistakenly detect the abundant new antibodies in response to the vaccine. Even then, the result will not be a false positive, but rather an inconclusive result and the person will later test negative.

AIDS pseudoscientists have also used cross-reactivity of HIV antibody tests to various other diseases to claim that there is a conspiracy behind the expansion of conditions that result in an AIDS diagnosis. For example, tuberculosis (TB) is now an AIDS-defining condition and cervical cancer was added to the definition of AIDS in 1993. Like the Perth Group, Duesberg associate Claus Kohnlein misuses clinically diagnosed AIDS to question the validity of HIV testing. For example, Kohnlein stated:

> By now about 30 afflictions all of which were known before, are being renamed to AIDS in the presence of a positive HIV-test. This also is not an increase of diseases of course – but just a redefinition. This circular definition HIV+/TB = AIDS and HIV−/TB = TB makes the correlation HIV–AIDS appear 100%. For example, a patient who suffers from TB and who is also HIV-positive is an AIDS patient today, and a woman who suffers from cervical carcinoma is an AIDS patient today, and a patient with a lymphoma is today not a lymphoma patient but also an AIDS patient if he has antibodies against HIV.[6]

Rebecca Culshaw's conspiracy theory also misuses AIDS diagnoses to argue against the validity of HIV test results:

> Some of the [AIDS] conditions listed are not even caused by immune deficiency, whereas others are clearly politically motivated, such as the 1993 inclusion of invasive cervical cancer. One can only presume that this disease was added to correct the disparity between male and female AIDS numbers, as there is little basis for including as 'AIDS-defining' a cancer that is relatively common among women with no evidence of immune suppression whatsoever.[7]

Neville Hodgkinson, who writes denialist columns for an online newsletter, also describes a conspiracy to find antibodies in people with AIDS:

… HIV pioneers found some 30 proteins in filtered material that gathered at a density characteristic of retroviruses. They attributed some of these to various parts of the virus. But they never demonstrated that these so-called "HIV antigens" belonged to a new retrovirus. So, out of the 30 proteins, how did they select the ones to be defined as being from HIV? The answer is shocking, and goes to the root of what is probably the biggest scandal in medical history. They selected those that were most reactive with antibodies in blood samples from AIDS patients and those at risk of AIDS. This means that "HIV" antigens are defined as such not on the basis of being shown to belong to HIV, but on the basis that they react with antibodies in AIDS patients. AIDS patients are then diagnosed as being infected with HIV on the basis that they have antibodies which react with those same antigens. The reasoning is circular.[8]

The very idea that HIV tests were developed as a means of explaining AIDS defies logic because a person who tests HIV positive today may not develop AIDS-related conditions for years. Two other preposterous propositions used to undermine HIV tests include the myth that HIV has not been "purified" and the deliberate confusion between HIV antibodies and the virus itself.

The Pure Virus Myth

Another ploy to discredit HIV antibody tests relies on the myth that HIV has never been purified. The myth goes that HIV has not been isolated in "pure" form, so there is no "gold standard" for the test. The pure virus myth is based on the false notion that HIV has never been "purified" to a state that would allow the test to detect antibodies against HIV without "contaminating proteins" from cells, ignoring the basic biology of viruses. When a virus erupts, or buds, from a cell it always carries elements from the cell itself. By definition, a virus uses the cell's machinery to produce more virus particles. There is no such thing as a virus that is completely pure, "uncontaminated" by cell proteins. Just as polio and herpes viruses that have been isolated and micrographed, so too has HIV. The demand that only "pure" virus can be the gold standard for an HIV test reflects either a poor understanding for what is required in virus isolation or a disregard for the biology of viruses.

Following the same flawed logic, Henry Bauer states that HIV is supposed to be a retrovirus: particles of RNA covered by protein. He says that to know what that RNA is, and what the viral proteins are, one would have to isolate them with "nothing else present." Bauer states that there has never been an isolated HIV particle from an HIV positive person shown by electron microscopy to be pure. Remarkably, he references two papers that have in fact isolated HIV and the virus isolates included mixtures of cellular proteins. Bauer nonsensically claims that the presence of the cellular proteins results in an impure virus. The basic flaw in his logic is that HIV tests do not detect viral proteins (antigens), but rather the tests detect proteins produced by the immune system (antibodies) to react against the virus. In the absence of an autoimmune disease, people do not produce antibodies against their own cellular proteins!

Bauer uses the pure virus myth to set up his bizarre notion that it is an abundance of antibodies in the blood of Africans and people of African heritage that cross-react with HIV tests. He explains why African-Americans and Africans are more likely to test HIV positive than whites and why dark-skinned Hispanics are more likely to test positive than light-skinned Hispanics. Bauer uses this wacky idea as the basis for his "analysis" of HIV testing data to "prove" that HIV tests do not relate to AIDS diagnoses. He actually claims that people with dark-skin have immune systems that fundamentally differ from light-skinned people and these differences explain why dark skinned people are more likely to test HIV positive, and why Hispanics have HIV prevalence somewhere between whites and African Americans, and why Hispanics of Caribbean heritage have higher HIV prevalence than Latin Americans. In his own words Bauer states:

> Humans evolved in Africa with dark skin for the optimum degree of sunshine-filtering. As humans migrated out of Africa into northern and temperate regions, more of the incident sunshine was needed in order to manufacture sufficient vitamin D, and so skin tones became lighter. As well as much sunshine, tropical regions also harbor a great variety of bacterial, microbial, parasitic, and viral diseases. It would therefore be curious if humans, evolving in Africa, had not acquired strong immune responses against a wide range of those challenges to health. As humans migrated to other, non-tropical parts of the world where challenges to the immune system were less frequent, it seems reasonable that the responses generated by the immune system might have become somewhat weakened.[9]

Needless to say, Bauer does not offer any evidence for genetic racial differences in immune system functioning that could lead to a false positive HIV test. Current science on race and immunology actually contradicts Bauer's treatise on race and immunity. As pointed out by Professor Wilmot James at the University of Cape Town, race differences in immune responses relate to geographic patterns of ancestry, not racial genetics. Hemoglobin S, for example, offers protection against malaria and specific immune cell characteristics protect against small pox. These protective mechanisms relate ancestral history to certain locales with prevalent diseases rather than to racial genetics. Research conducted by Professor Eileen Dolan at the University of Chicago confirms that there are such differences in immune responses to bacteria and these differences may explain how populations differ in vulnerability to disease and drug toxicities, such as medication side-effects. But the research does not suggest that Africans have more antibodies than non-Africans or that such antibodies would confuse an HIV test.

The pure virus myth and its associated claims are bogus because HIV, like all viruses, depends on its host cell to replicate new virus particles. Researchers who study isolates of HIV and its proteins, including those very scientists that Henry Bauer himself cites, clearly debunk the pure virus myth by concluding that HIV subverts cellular processes to facilitate its own replication.[10]

Everyone Is HIV Positive

Journalist Celia Farber confuses HIV infection with antibody responses when she states that all babies born to HIV positive mothers are born HIV positive and that most become negative months later. She creates the false impression of erroneous HIV test results because it is the tragic but indisputable fact that HIV infected babies cannot possibly become HIV uninfected. In this respect, Farber is suggesting that all babies born to women with HIV/AIDS have HIV infection. Women do pass on their antibodies to their babies, a natural mechanism that protects newborns from disease. However, the child's body eliminates the mother's antibodies within 18 months from birth and usually sooner. Of course, if a baby is truly infected with HIV, it produces its own persistent antibodies, so if a child is still antibody positive when 18 months old, he or she is most certainly infected with HIV. Without antiretroviral treatment, one in three babies born to HIV infected women will have HIV infection. With antiretroviral treatment for both the mother and baby, the percentage is reduced to nearly zero.

Given the stark statistic of one in three babies born to untreated HIV positive mothers also becoming infected, it is easy to understand how dangerous and damaging misinformation can be. AIDS pseudoscience undermines HIV testing because it leads to obvious questions such as "If HIV does not cause infection, why take the test?" and "If the test result is invalid, why bother testing?" People, including pregnant women, may not take the test and those who test HIV positive may disregard the result. Texas college math professor Rebecca Culshaw actually recommends that people not bother testing for HIV, drawing this ill-informed conclusion:

> I cannot buy the idea that any individual needs to have a diagnostic HIV test. A negative test may not be accurate (whatever that means), but a positive one can create utter havoc and destruction in a person's life – all for a virus that most likely does absolutely nothing. I do not feel it is going too far to say that these tests ought to be banned for diagnostic purposes.[11]

The most perverse case of pseudo-immunology comes from nutritionist Roberto Giraldo. Antibody tests, such as the HIV test, require a standard protocol that involves diluting blood to reduce concentrations of blood serum to a constant level. To perform the test properly and get a valid result, the blood sample must be properly prepared. While working in a New York medical laboratory, Giraldo took it upon himself to answer the dubious question "What makes HIV so unique that the test serum needs to be diluted 400 times? And what would happen if the individual's serum is not diluted?" Giraldo's bizarre question reminds me of when my 5-year-old daughter asked what would happen if we made pancakes without adding milk. Should we expect pancakes? In reporting his bizarre pseudoscientific experiment, Giraldo wrote the following:

> To answer these questions I ran an experiment in a medical laboratory in Yorktown Heights, New York. I ran it using the same test kit reagents that are usually used to run the ELISA test in most clinical laboratories worldwide. I first took samples of blood that, at 1:400 dilution, tested negative for antibodies to HIV. I then ran the exact same serum samples through the test again, but this time without diluting them. Tested straight, they all came positive.
>
> Since that time, I have run about 100 specimens and have always gotten the same result. I even ran my own blood which, at 1:400, reacts negative. At 1:1 [undiluted] it reacted positive. I should mention that with the exception of my own blood, the patient samples all came from doctors who requested HIV tests. It is therefore likely that most of the blood samples that I tested belonged to individuals at risk for AIDS.[12]

This bogus experiment was published in the now defunct magazine *Continuum*, created as an outlet for AIDS pseudoscience, which by the way had the sole purpose of circumventing peer review. Other AIDS pseudoscientists propagate Giraldo's myth that everyone tests HIV positive by repeating his erroneous findings as if they were actual science. This strange and unethical experiment has become a fixture in the anti-HIV testing lore of pseudoscience and denialism.

The upshot of pseudo-immunology thus far is that, like pseudo-virology, the belief that HIV does not even exist. The HIV test is reacting to who knows what proteins, and people are diagnosed with an infection that they simply do not have. This brand of pseudoscience allows denialists to conclude that HIV tests are a fraud. A second genre of pseudo-immunologists do accept the existence of the virus, they just claim that it is harmless.

Pseudo-immunology II: HIV Does Not Cause AIDS

Most AIDS pseudoscience is rooted in Peter Duesberg's assertion that HIV is a harmless virus that does not and cannot cause AIDS. Actually, what they are saying is that the virus is a victim that "has been wrongly accused of committing the AIDS crime."[13] However, true followers of Duesberg do not dispute the existence of HIV or AIDS. They do dispute though the causal connection between HIV and AIDS. Just as Duesberg questions whether a single gene can cause cancer, he poses the question "How can one tiny virus be the cause of so many diseases?" This erroneous belief is the basis for much of President Mbeki's South African AIDS policy, which was at least in part based on the notion that a single virus could never cause so many diseases. To think that HIV science says that HIV causes many diseases is simply wrong. HIV causes one disease – the systematic destruction of the immune system – which then opens the door to the myriad of diseases that we call AIDS. Simply stated, the virus kills immune cells which leaves the body vulnerable to many diseases, any of which will signal the onset of full-blown AIDS.

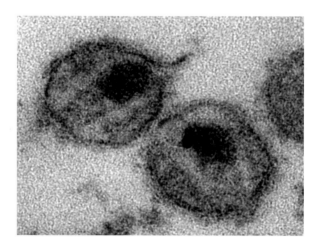

Photo 3.1 This thin-section transmission electron micrograph (TEM) depicted the ultrastructural details of two HIV particles.
Source: Centers for Disease Control and Prevention, http://phil.cdc.gov/phil/details.asp

If one adheres to Duesberg's view that HIV does not cause AIDS, one must ask what does? Eleni Papadopulos-Eleopulos of the Perth Group takes the position that AIDS results from lifestyle choices. Specifically, she says that immune destruction happens when homosexuals are exposed to nitrites and anally deposited semen, when drug abusers are exposed to opiates and nitrites and when hemophiliacs receive contaminated blood clotting factors. Her twisted conclusion falls right in line with Duesberg's and she goes further to claim "potent oxidizing agents" ultimately cause AIDS. There is, of course, no evidence that semen, illicit drugs, malnutrition, poor drinking water, HIV treatments, stress, the sun, having a common cold, or other immune suppressors deplete CD4/T-Helper cells, damage the immune system, and cause AIDS.

Selecting a single sentence from a single study is how Duesberg himself has reasserted that HIV does not cause AIDS. In an interview with *City on a Hill Press*, the reporter paraphrases and quotes him as shown here:

> HIV cannot even be found in AIDS patients. 'There is no viral load, only antibodies,' said Duesberg. 'The load is generated on the bench by the scientist.' In contrast, conventional pathogenic viruses are abundant and antibodies have not yet neutralized them. He points to recent research in the *Journal of the American Medical Association (JAMA)* done by Rodriguez, et al. from 2006, in which 'viral load' had no correlation with AIDS. HIV 'RNA loads are high, low, or undetectable in asymptomatic carriers of AIDS.'[14]

Duesberg misuses the concluding sentence, in fact, turns its meaning on its head. Rodriguez and colleagues actually showed that the initial viral load that HIV/AIDS patients have when they enter clinical care does not itself predict declines in CD4/T-Helper cells as expected. The authors never imply that HIV does not cause AIDS or that viral load is not associated with AIDS. As one of the study's authors told me, the findings in the paper in no way suggest that HIV does not cause AIDS. What the study *does* suggest is that HIV viral load alone does not accurately predict or sufficiently explain CD4/T-cell decline. Part of the problem is that there is a lot of individual variation in the loss of CD4/T-cells in people with HIV/AIDS. The scientific point made by Rodriguez et al. is that there may be several important factors affecting the decline of CD4/T-cells. However, all of the factors under consideration directly contribute to HIV infection – including HIV proteins in the lymph nodes that kill the cells. Concerned about the misuse of their research by Duesberg, Culshaw and a host of other AIDS pseudoscientists, Rodriguez and his co-authors wrote an explanation of their findings that included the following:

> There is absolutely no doubt that HIV is the cause of AIDS; far from challenging the veracity of this statement, our work further confirms it. This is easily appreciated from our initial analysis of the data, which shows that on average, individuals with higher viral loads tend to lose CD4 cells more rapidly than those with lower viral loads. There is no contradiction between this finding and our main message, because the overall trend among a group of subjects cannot be directly translated into a prediction of what will happen to a single individual within that group. Importantly, this finding replicates, rather than disputes, the substance of the seminal paper by Mellors et al (Ann Internal Med 1997; 126: 946–954), which demonstrated this almost 10 years ago. Thus, using our work to claim that those previous conclusions are invalid reveals either a combination of sloppy thinking, sloppy reading or malicious intent. We choose to believe that it is the first two.[15]

Another example of pseudo-immunology comes from the Alberta Reappraising AIDS Society. Amidst his other pseudoscientific articles, David Crowe claims that the National Institutes of Health (NIH) cannot account for what causes AIDS. He states that the NIH has created a "nice graph" depicting how HIV causes AIDS but supplies "no data" to support the graph. I presented this same graph in Chapter 2 to illustrate the relationship between HIV viral load, CD4/T-helper cells, and AIDS (see Fig. 2.7). This HIV disease process, or pathogenesis, graph represents the accumulation of years of research, never intending to depict the results of any single study. However, because the graph uses dots and squares for markers on the lines, Crowe says that the graph intends to represent a "real study," revealing a conspiracy plot in the NIH aimed at discrediting Peter Duesberg.[16] It is nearly impossible to follow Crowe's logic in unfolding the conspiracy behind the graph, and that of course is the point. Anyone who is questioning the cause of AIDS will be more confused after reading his convoluted account than they were before.

Proof that HIV Does Not Cause AIDS

Duesberg is not the only seriously credentialed academic to take up a pseudo-immunological approach to AIDS. Henry Bauer – Professor Emeritus of Chemistry and Science Studies and Dean Emeritus of Arts and Sciences at the respected Virginia Polytechnic Institute and State University – uses HIV testing data and statistical analysis of AIDS diagnoses to show that HIV cannot cause AIDS. Bauer bases his conclusions on the erroneous use of HIV testing data and AIDS diagnoses. He misuses the established fact that it takes 10 years for people who test HIV positive to develop AIDS. His misuse comes in the form of his mixing and matching sources of HIV testing and cases of AIDS that have absolutely no relationship at all. Then he reports that his analysis shows that results from HIV tested military recruits in the early 1980s, for example, do not correspond to the US AIDS diagnoses 10 years later. On this basis, he claims that he has proven that HIV cannot cause AIDS! He also claims that HIV cannot be transmitted sexually because women military recruits are just as likely as men to test HIV positive, and yet men in the United States are far more likely to develop AIDS. In his own words:

> HIV is neither sexually transmitted nor increasingly prevalent. HIV and AIDS are not correlated geographically. HIV and AIDS are not correlated chronologically. HIV and AIDS are not correlated in their relative impact on women and men. Nor are HIV and AIDS correlated in their relative impact on white and black people. HIV is necessary but insufficient to cause AIDS.[17]

This is obviously the proof that denialists have been waiting for. David Crowe "reviewed" *The Origins, Persistence, and Failings of HIV/AIDS Theory* prior to publication, constituting what would seem to be true peer review, in pseudoscience that is. Crowe personally recommended the book, especially for Bauer's "innovative use of statistics and resolution of race differences in AIDS." Rebecca Culshaw also relies on Bauer's analysis, stating that "in this devastating analysis, Bauer points out many of the epidemiological aspects of HIV that are literally incompatible with the hypotheses that it causes AIDS."[18] Internet blogger Darin Brown stated, the book "not only presents novel scientific arguments against the HIV/AIDS hypothesis, he also uses his experience in science studies to provide a compelling response to the frequent semi-rhetorical question, 'How could so many scientists be so wrong?'"[19] Anthony Brink, South African attorney said that the book was incredibly important for its careful analysis. William F. Shughart of the University of Mississippi stated that Bauer should be commended for "Skillfully collating, summarizing and analyzing an extensive literature, including hundreds of scientific studies, published and unpublished, reports produced by government agencies and non-government organizations, and statements issued by public-health experts, Bauer methodically undermines every argument and stylized fact ostensibly linking AIDS to HIV."[20]

These endorsements of Bauer's wacky book speak volumes about how AIDS pseudoscience is self-perpetuated and how pseudoscience fuels denialism. Bauer has never done AIDS research. In fact, he has never done any scientific research. Henry Bauer is a pseudoscientist's pseudoscientist! A leader in the world of the strange and unusual, he is the former editor of the *Journal of Scientific Exploration*, the major outlet for studies in UFOlogy, paranormal activity, extrasensory powers, alien abductions, etc. He has presented his AIDS analyses at the annual conference of the Society of Scientific Exploration, along side such work as "Anomalous Energies and Balls of Light in Crop Circles," "UFO research: Where Do We Go From Here?," and "Consciousness, Psi, and the Two Brains."

Henry Bauer is also one of the world's leading authorities on the Loch Ness Monster. That is right, the Loch Ness Monster! In one of his most known works on Nessies published in the *Journal of Scientific Exploration,* he wrote:

On my ninth visit to Loch Ness, I no longer expect to see the monster, even though I fully believe that it exists. Others may think that paradoxical, but I think it shows that I have learned a bit about the Monster, and about some other things as well. In 1958, on my first visit and as a casual tourist, I didn't expect to see the Monster because I didn't believe in it. In fact, I actively disbelieved in it. I knew the Monster to be a myth, a joke, or a hoax, good for the tourist trade but not for serious consideration. So I gave a mental sneer when, browsing in the library a few years later, I came upon a book entitled Loch Ness Monster. Superciliously I riffled the pages and found some glossy ones with photos, and those photos gave me pause. A long pause, for I took the book home and read it, and – for perhaps the first time in my life – I really didn't know what to believe.[21]

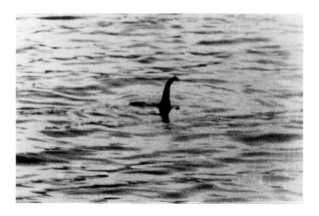

Photo 3.2 The mythical Loch Ness Monster
Source: Getty Images

Bauer is obviously serious about stretching the boundaries of science. Perhaps among the most curious enigmas in the world of denialism is finding the likes of him in the halls of academia. He is a tenured professor at a respected research institution. Undoubtedly, Bauer's interests in the strange fringes of science made him a colorful character on the Virginia Tech campus. I would imagine that some undergraduate students were mesmerized by his stories of tracking down Nessies in the fogging waters of Loch Ness. As I was told, I do not doubt that he was a competent administrator as well. Still, it would be hard to believe that he was ever taken seriously by his colleagues given that he had not conducted scientific research and delved deeply into the world of pseudoscience. It may be that he was unbothered by any professional disrespect given his views on the narrow mindedness of the scientific ortho-doxy. With AIDS, however, Bauer fully expects to be taken seriously.

In one of his several but similarly flawed analyses, Bauer compares HIV testing data from military recruits in the 1980s, who represented young people from across the United States but were not even remotely representa-tive of people at risk for HIV/AIDS, to US AIDS cases a decade later. For the most part, military recruits could not be any more different from the subpopulations most affected by AIDS. In fact, the military systematically excludes from service the groups that are at greatest risk for HIV/AIDS, namely gay men and injection drug users. Surely, there are gay men and drug users in the military, but only when they go unnoticed. So epidemiolo-gically speaking, the universe of young recruits is significantly skewed in the opposite direction from the populations that were subsequently diagno-sed with AIDS. Moreover, military recruits over-represent people in rural America and under-represent urban areas where HIV/AIDS is most prevalent. Most military recruits are under age 25 whereas HIV infections occur throughout young adulthood. Bauer claims HIV cannot cause AIDS because the demographics of people who have tested positive for HIV in the military are not like those who develop AIDS. He also notes that the frequency of testing HIV positive varies between military recruits and job corps applicants, concluding that HIV is present more in lower social strata. Although this fact is widely known, Bauer twists it to confirm his thesis that HIV tests are invalid. The analysis defies logic.

Amazingly, extrapolating military HIV testing data from the 1980s to predict AIDS in the United States was not even Henry Bauer's original idea. In 1992, ultra-conservative journalist and Duesberg sympathizer Tom Bethell noted that "Routine testing of army recruits shows the HIV-positive percentage of the population has remained constant since 1985, and AIDS remains largely confined to risk groups-homosexuals and drug-users. Neither finding is consistent with a new virus spreading in the population."[22] Bauer seems to have built his argument on Bethell's crude attempt to line up HIV testing in military recruits with national AIDS cases.

Bauer also concludes that HIV is not transmitted sexually because the AIDS epidemic does not look in any way like epidemics of gonorrhea and syphilis. A college junior in computer sciences who attended one of Henry Bauer's lectures was even able to point out the flawed logic. The student said Bauer's comparing HIV to two bacterial infections was a "fundamentally bad analysis," like comparing "apples and gerbils." Viral infections like HIV cannot be cured and have completely different epidemiologic outlooks from bacterial infections, such as gonorrhea and syphilis. Bauer responded to the student by saying "maybe I should use Hepatitis B [a viral infection] as a comparison. I haven't looked at it specifically."[23] In fact, this college junior demonstrated a far superior understanding of epidemiology than Bauer. The scientific point is easily illustrated by looking at how HIV does correspond to another sexually transmitted viral infection, like Herpes Simplex Virus, particularly in places where both infections are epidemic, like Africa. Figure 3.1 shows that Herpes Simplex Virus infection does in fact track closely to HIV infection in men and women in Kenya and Zambia. Both HIV and Herpes Simplex Virus have a strong co-occurrence in men and women throughout adolescence and early adulthood.

Bauer also claims that people with hemophilia should have never been included in AIDS statistics because hemophilia itself is immune suppressing, stating that it is possible that Ryan White, who was diagnosed in 1984 at age 13 and died of AIDS in 1990, could have contracted HIV from a source other than blood products used in treating hemophilia. And Bauer posed as a question another possibility:

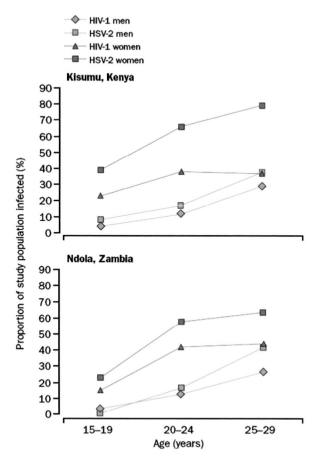

Fig. 3.1 The co-occurring epidemics of HIV and Herpes Simplex Virus (HSV-2) for men and women in two sub-Saharan African cities
Source: Schmid et al. 2004

> Poor Ryan White had indeed been born in very ill health for a long time on account of his severe hemophilia. Testing for HIV just introduced in 1984 – perhaps he might have been HIV positive at birth? It is possible that his death was hastened by HIV medications? [24]

Table 3.1 shows some more examples of Bauer's faulty logic and wrong conclusions. It is not so remarkable that Bauer has contributed to AIDS pseudoscience, given his long and strange career. Bauer had hoped that his book would land him an interview on the Today Show and change the course of AIDS research and treatments. What is most remarkable about Bauer is how rapidly denialism has embraced him and taken up his conclusions. Bauer offers a vivid example of how denialism indiscriminately embraces anything that agrees with it.

Table 3.1 Flawed logic and incorrect conclusions about AIDS highlighted by Henry Bauer

Henry Bauer's conclusion	Scientific reality
Frequency of HIV positive tests for TB patients is about the same as, perhaps even higher than, for STI clinic patients. That makes no sense if HIV is contracted sexually.	TB is an opportunistic infection, becoming active in people with immune suppression. It stands to reason that TB patients have a high prevalence of HIV infection. The HIV–TB co-epidemics are well established.
Those visiting STI clinics and not specifically HIV clinics presumably know that their behavior may have exposed them to syphilis or gonorrhea but also believe that they did not put themselves at risk for HIV. And yet HIV among STI patients and HIV clinics is quite similar.	This is an absurd conclusion seeing as ALL patients at any HIV clinic will be HIV positive but only a proportion of people at any STI clinic will be infected with HIV.
Patients in hospitals because of illnesses unrelated to HIV are about 10 times more likely to have HIV than generally healthy populations such as people in the military – and even 100 times greater repeat blood donors.	People with HIV encounter serious health challenges that require hospitalization, even if not an AIDS defining condition. HIV impacts the nervous system, the vascular system, and the digestive system. So a person with HIV may be hospitalized for dehydration due to excessive diarrhea, but the visit will not be attributed directly to HIV. And, there is no population with lower HIV infection rates than repeat blood donors given that they have undergone repeated screening for HIV.
Prostitutes should be at high risk for HIV. Yet a European study found that only 1.5% of prostitutes who did not use drugs had HIV, while 32% of those who did use drugs had HIV. Which then is the risky behavior, sex or drugs?	In a low HIV prevalence place, such as much of Europe and the US, prostitutes are at higher risk for HIV by injecting drugs than unprotected sex. But there are raging sexually transmitted HIV epidemics among prostitutes in countries with high HIV prevalence, such as much of southern Africa where there is little drug abuse.

Source for Bauer's logic, Henry Bauer (2007), *The Origins, Persistence, and Failings of HIV/AIDS Theory.*
Note: STI, Sexually Transmitted Infections.

From Giraldo's belief that HIV does not exist, to Duesberg's claim that HIV is harmless, to Bauer's analysis that shows HIV tests are invalid, AIDS pseudoscience flies in the face of 25 years of AIDS science. HIV has been isolated, micrographed, and studied. HIV antibodies are specific and detected by HIV tests. HIV causes the same single disease in everyone infected, namely the systematic destruction of the immune system. Once its toll is taken, the immune system collapses, giving way to a cascade of diseases, any of which will signal full-blown AIDS. The AIDS pseudosciences reviewed thus far are easily refuted by the medical facts of the disease. In a step closer to reality, there are pseudoscientists who point to the importance of co-factors in the development of AIDS.

Pseudo-immunology III: HIV Is Necessary but Insufficient to Cause AIDS

Not all AIDS pseudoscientists agree with Duesberg's claim that HIV is a harmless passenger virus. Some have stated that HIV plays a role in AIDS but is too "weak" to cause AIDS by itself. Many factors can facilitate the progression of HIV disease, such as alcohol, drug abuse, smoking, numerous infections, and conditions of poverty. So-called co-factors stimulate the immune system and activate CD4/T-Helper cells, which in turn trigger HIV replication, and therefore accelerate HIV disease progression. In the early 1980s, it was perfectly reasonable to hold the position that AIDS was the result of multiple competing factors.[25] AIDS pseudoscientists falsely claim, however, that without co-factors, HIV alone cannot cause AIDS. One of the early proponents of the co-factor theory of AIDS was the Robert Root-Bernstein, Professor of Life Sciences at Michigan State University. Root-Bernstein published a book in 1993 *Rethinking AIDS: The Tragic Cost of Premature Consensus*, in which he claimed that HIV is insufficient to cause AIDS. As AIDS science advanced, respected scientist Root-Bernstein softened his views. He is now critical of those who follow Duesberg to argue that HIV is harmless.[26]

Those who believe that HIV is insufficient to cause AIDS encourage people to make lifestyle changes in order to avoid the disease while also discouraging the use of antiretroviral medications. Eating a balanced diet, reducing stress, avoiding new infections, and so forth offer great health benefits for people infected with HIV. However, there is no evidence that these kinds of changes in lifestyle help people with HIV to evade AIDS.

A Closer Look at Poverty, Africa, and AIDS

An unbiased look at the relationship between poverty and AIDS shows that it is ridiculous to conclude that poverty itself is the cause of this disease. In New York State, for example, more than one in five children live in poverty, as do one in five 19–60 year olds as well as persons over 60. Poverty rates obviously do not mirror AIDS diagnoses in New York, where the vast majority of AIDS occurs in young adults and poverty is evenly distributed across ages. It is also the case that more Hispanics in New York live in poverty than do blacks and whites. Despite these differences in poverty, most people with HIV/AIDS in New York are black.

Does poverty account for AIDS in Africa? As discussed in Chapter 2, the poorest countries in the world often have among the lowest number of people affected by AIDS, as shown in Table 2.1. Economist Nicoli Nattrass at the University of Cape Town has shown that African countries are as much as 18 times more burdened by AIDS than other developing countries with comparable or even more severe poverty. And in Africa, some of the more developed countries, particularly South Africa, carry the greatest AIDS burden. When people who have AIDS from neighboring countries seek refuge in South Africa, their AIDS does not go away suddenly with cleaner water and more food. Another false conclusion drawn by Duesberg and others is that the fact of devastating illness and death caused by AIDS in Africa is refutable because Africa continues to enjoy positive population growth. Duesberg asks, "Since 1984 black Africa has grown from about 400 to now 650 million! So – where is the new decimating epidemic?"[27] Countries throughout southern Africa have suffered severe decreases in life expectancy over the years that coincide with AIDS, as shown in Fig. 3.2. Life expectancies that were improving during the post-colonial years of the 1960s and 1970s began to erode in the 1980s and 1990s, and life expectancy in many countries is now worse than even during the 1950s, the last full decade of colonialism.

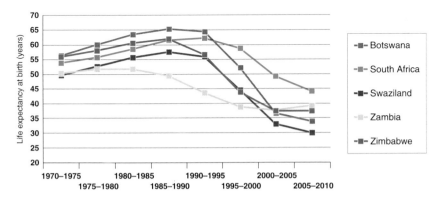

Fig. 3.2 Changes in life expectancies in African countries with the highest rates of AIDS
Source: United Nations Population Division (2004). World Population Prospects: The 2004 Revision, database

The reason why some countries afflicted by AIDS sustain positive population growth is simply high birth rates. In eastern Zimbabwe, for example, Gregson and colleagues at the Imperial College of London studied population changes between the years 1995 and 2005. The life expectancy in rural areas of Zimbabwe declined by more than 20 years since 1998. HIV/AIDS has reduced population growth by two-thirds in much of Zimbabwe, but the overall population growth remains unchanged, at about 1% annually. Gregson concluded that HIV/AIDS has had "devastating effects on countries like Zimbabwe, but in terms of demographic impact, it has not had as much of an impact as some of the most pessimistic estimates. . . .Our research shows that, in spite of countless people having lost their lives to the virus, more people are still being born than are dying."[28] Duesberg is right to say that population growth remains positive in some places in Africa. But he is wrong – and I would suggest deceitful – to say that this trend raises questions about the devastation that HIV/AIDS has wrought on this region of the world.

Pseudo-pharmacology: HIV Treatments Are Toxic Poison

So there are many pseudoscientific explanations of the causes of HIV/AIDS. Not surprisingly as it turns out, there is pseudoscience surrounding the issue of treatment as well. In the 1980s, the drug zidovudine (AZT) was the only treatment available for HIV infection. At the time, high doses of AZT caused serious side-effects. While it suppressed HIV replication and slowed HIV disease, it did so for only a short time. One problem was that no one knew then what dose to use and so doctors used more drug than may have been necessary to suppress the virus. A second problem was that HIV can rapidly mutate when only one type of antiretroviral medication is used, allowing the virus to develop genetic resistance. Comparing today's HIV treatments, which include combinations of multiple medications, to AZT alone is like comparing the Ford Model T to a Ford Mustang. The evidence that antiretroviral medications slow HIV disease and that people who take these drugs live longer and healthier lives is undeniable. On a population level, we can see that people with AIDS who receive treatment are living longer healthier lives than ever before. Unlike all other causes of death among young adults, AIDS deaths climbed dramatically during the 1980s and early 1990s. Since 1996, when combination therapies were introduced on a wide-scale, results have been dramatic: not only have AIDS deaths declined, the number of HIV/AIDS-related hospitalizations has plummeted. In fact, hospital beds once allocated specifically for AIDS patients no longer exist. People living with

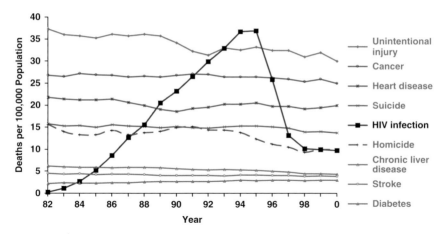

Fig. 3.3 Changes in leading causes of death among US young adults, ages 25–45
Source: Centers for Disease Control and Prevention

HIV/AIDS have returned to work in droves. As shown in Fig. 3.3 combina-tions of HIV medications that became available in 1996 led to an indisputable reversal in AIDS deaths in the United States.

Only a denialist could deny the overwhelming evidence for the benefits of antiretroviral medications. Duesberg claims that the shift in AIDS deaths follows the path predicted by declining drug use a decade earlier. However, he contradicts his own premise that antiretroviral medications cause AIDS. That is, why are there fewer people with AIDS after the medications become available? The only explanation for the reduction in AIDS deaths is the increased availability of HIV treatments. The same contradiction occurs in Duesberg's theory of cancer, where he says carcinogens in the environment cause abnormal chromosomes, which in turn are "the cause of cancer." In fact, a paper presented at his own Aneuploidy conference showed data from over 100 years in Germany that determined there were no changes in cancer deaths despite increases in environmental toxins. The same pattern is appar-ent in a briefer period shown in Fig. 3.3, where cancer deaths remain stable over the years that AIDS deaths change dramatically.

In another example of science misuse, Duesberg stated that, "Hundreds of investigators just published in the *Lancet* the largest epidemiological survey of its kind. The conclusion was 'Virological response after starting HAART [combination ARV therapy] improved over calendar years, but such improvement has not translated into decrease in mortality."[29] Con-trary to Duesberg's selective use of the study, the results never call into question the life-extending value of antiretroviral medications in treating HIV infection. The reasons why medications worked less well in the later years of the study was simply because the patients included in the study changed over time. More people with tuberculosis (TB) were in the study in its later years and TB is among the most lethal AIDS-related conditions. The study actually concluded that early diagnosis and treatment (of HIV) is of great importance to prevent clinical progression of HIV.[30] Once again it is Duesberg's exploitation and warping of science that is most angering.

There are numerous examples of less sophisticated, although no less destructive, manipulations of HIV treatment research in the interest of denialism. Some of them verge into paranoid and conspiratorial theories about the disease and how to treat it. Some AIDS pseudoscientists have led the charge that promoting the idea that HIV medication programs are part of a global conspiracy between the pharmaceutical companies, the Bill and Melinda Gates Foundation, former US President Bill Clinton, Irish musician Bono, the National Institutes of Health, the World Health Organization, and the CIA, all working together to sell medications to the world's poor. For example, Duesberg's collaborator David Rasnick in his contributions to the 2000 South African Presidential panel on AIDS stated,

> I don't have to point out to the government of South Africa that the involvement of the FBI, CIA, and NSA in AIDS represents a far greater threat to our democracies than to HIV. The most astounding thing to me about all of this is that the greatest threat to our democracies has turned out not to be goose-stepping soldiers in camouflage but rather the chronic fear peddled by white-coated scientists and physicians and their sycophants in the media who have squandered billions of dollars of taxpayers' money annually.[31]

Matthias Rath, the German entrepreneur who sells vitamins to treat AIDS, also sees a global conspiracy to promote HIV medications and he says that Bill Gates is personally monitoring his activities:

> The equation is simple: the end of the AIDS business with disease will destroy the entire credibility of the pharmaceutical industry and will terminate the drug investment business worldwide. The collapse of this multi-billion dollar investment business, in turn, will lead to a major crisis in the whole investment industry. In other words, the 'Mother Theresa' PR-stunt of Bill Gates is a desperate, self-serving activity trying to stop this meltdown. If Gates is not successful, and the AIDS genocide by the drug cartel is ended, then the whole paper-wealth of Billy Gates is worthless.[32]

Conspiracy thinking spans across the spectrum of denialism. In 2000, President Thabo Mbeki of South Africa expressed his own conspiracy concerns to the African National Congress members of parliament saying,

> If we say HIV equals AIDS then we must say equals drugs. Pharmaceutical companies want to sell drugs which they can't do unless HIV causes AIDS, so they don't want this thesis to be attacked. That's one problem. The other one is the international political environment where the CIA has got involved. So, the US says we will give loans to Africa to pay for US drugs.[33]

AIDS pseudoscientists also use campaigns of fear and conspiracy-mongering to attack HIV treatments. One technique is to emphasize the negative side-effects without acknowledging any benefits. Medications are "toxic" and "poison." Doctors are portrayed as coercing their patients into taking medications. Denialist journalist Celia Farber even claims that there is an entire "surveillance system in place to ensure that people stick to the new drugs despite side-effects. Computer chips are embedded in bottle caps that record the date and time of each opening. Beepers, support groups, buddy systems, AIDS professionals that infiltrate people's social networks."[34] She is of course implying a vast conspiracy, but is really referring to the strategies used to help people to remember to take their pills. It would appear to be the "don't forget to take your pills conspiracy."

Perhaps most tragically, AIDS pseudoscientists use the same illogic to argue against using medications to prevent HIV transmission from pregnant women to their unborn babies. Since 1996, we know that AZT reduces the risk for transmitting HIV from mothers to newborns, from around one in three without treatments to nearly zero with treatments. But some women have refused to use AZT after hearing the rhetoric of AIDS pseudoscientists. Christine Maggiore, for example, denied that she was HIV infected and refused to take steps to protect her children from HIV infection. (As described in Chapter 1, the record shows that her daughter died of AIDS complications at the age of 3 years.) Sophie Brassard is another mother who refused HIV treatment for herself and for her children because she believed that the medications were harmful. Influenced by Maggiore's denialist organization Alive and Well and Duesberg, Brassard's sons became ill and she ultimately lost custody. Sophie Brassard died of AIDS complications in 2002.

In South Africa, HIV treatments have not been widely dispensed to pregnant women because of the influence of AIDS pseudoscience on the health ministry. Some one in five babies of HIV infected mothers in South Africa are born infected with HIV. To prove the point, McCord hospital in South Africa did institute combination treatments to prevent pregnant women from passing the virus to their babies and demonstrated only 3% of the babies born became infected. Still, many areas of South Africa have limited preventive treatment available and many women refused treatment because they trusted the recommendations of their health minister. By comparison, in Botswana, a much poorer country than South Africa, only 4% of babies born to infected mothers are infected with HIV since the country instituted universal testing and treatment of pregnant women. As shown in Fig. 3.4, in 1997 in New York State there were 97 HIV infected babies born compared to 18 in 2000 and just 10 in 2006. This decline occurred despite ever-increasing numbers of women infected with HIV. The only explanation for these life saving changes is the use of antiretroviral medications to prevent mother-to-child HIV transmission.

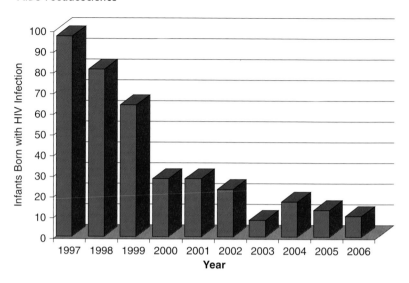

Fig. 3.4 Trends in HIV infected infants in New York State.
Source: New York State Department of Health

Denialism has also impeded the treatment of HIV infected children. For example, in some instances HIV treatment of children had been stopped after the false claims were made that HIV medications are harmful. In 2004 in New York City, Liam Scheff wrote a story on the Internet about children orphaned by AIDS receiving medications through a National Institutes of Health-funded clinical trial. The mainstream press picked up the story. The Traditional Values Coalition said, "Powerless and parentless children . . . are being scrutinized by the 'scientists' of the NIH. But using HIV-infected foster children, some as young as infants, for their AIDS experiments is beyond despicable. . . . these voiceless little ones have no rights and no one to speak for them when the NIH is in charge."[35] The situation escalated with the media becoming involved as well as child protection groups and ultimately some of the children were removed from treatment.

Pseudo-epidemiology: HIV Is Not Sexually Transmitted

Epidemiology is the study of factors that influence illness and health in populations, including the spread of disease. The science leaves no doubt about the sexual transmission of HIV, specifically including its transmission through vaginal sex. Studies that repeatedly interview couples where one person is HIV infected and their spouse or partner is not infected, document the routes of HIV transmission. Nothing can account for AIDS in Africa other than a heterosexual HIV epidemic.

In a classic example of how denialism can twist a single scientific finding to assert a false claim, one need not look any further than the myth that HIV is not heterosexually transmitted. Pseudoscientists continually misquote the research of Nancy Padian and her studies of heterosexual couples. Currently at the Research Triangle Institute, Padian is among the most recognized and respected AIDS epidemiologists in the world. Her research is continuously funded by the NIH and she has conducted very high profile research funded by the Bill and Melinda Gates Foundation. These credentials likely make her and her work open season for denialism. In one particular study, Padian set out to learn about couples in which one partner has HIV and other does not. In her acclaimed research, she took steps to prevent HIV transmission, particularly providing counseling and condoms to all of the couples in her study. Despite the clarity of her findings, there are countless examples of how AIDS pseudoscientists exploit Padian's research:

- In an open letter regarding a major research study conducted in South Africa, attorney Anthony Brink wrote: 'the largest and longest study of the heterosexual transmission of HIV in the United States', epidemiologist Dr Nancy Padian PhD and her colleagues .... that 'male-to-female per contact infectivity was estimated to be 0.0009'.....In sum, 'the largest and longest study of the heterosexual transmission of HIV in the United States' provides no evidence that HIV is sexually transmitted – instead, it adduces evidence that it isn't.[36]
- In her 2006 *Discover Magazine* interview, Celia Farber said "and one of the studies that the so-called dissidents have been drawing attention to is a study by a Berkeley researcher named Nancy Padian. Her study looked at transmission between couples where one was positive and one was negative. They had unprotected sex. They watched them over a period of 10 years. And there was not one single transmission in the whole group [during the 10-year study] – not one."[37]
- The Perth Group has repeatedly misused the Padian study, typically saying that there is no evidence that heterosexual sex could transmit the virus even if it does exist, which they say it surely does not.[38]
- The HEAL Toronto group stated that a 10 year study of sexual partners (one HIV+, one HIV–) recorded NO cases of sexual transmission. This same study concluded that it would take about 1,000 instances of heterosexual intercourse to transmit HIV once.[39]
- Henry Bauer stated that "It is also a shibboleth, and again also a myth, that unprotected intercourse brings great danger of spreading HIV. The risk of

sexual transmission of HIV has been found in several independent studies to be well under 1%, more like 0.1% or even less. . . . in a 10-year study, rather less than 1 per 1000 for male-to-female transmission (0.0009 was the actual figure) and much less than that (0.00011) for female-to-male transmission."[40]

Other than Robert Gallo's first isolation of HIV in 1984, no study has been as misrepresented by AIDS pseudoscientists as Nancy Padian's research has. Ultimately, Padian was compelled to explain her results with a direct appeal to ignore pseudoscience:

> HIV is unquestionably transmitted through heterosexual intercourse. Indeed, heterosexual intercourse is now responsible for 70–80% of all HIV transmissions worldwide. . . . the evidence for the sexual transmission of HIV is well documented, conclusive, and based on the standard, uncontroversial methods and practices of medical science. Individuals who cite the 1997 Padian et al. publication or data from other studies by our research group in an attempt to substantiate the myth that HIV is not transmitted sexually are ill informed, at best. Their misuse of these results is misleading, irresponsible, and potentially injurious to the public.
>
> A common practice is to quote out of context a sentence from the Abstract of the 1997 paper: "Infectivity for HIV through heterosexual transmission is low." Anyone who takes the trouble to read and understand the paper should appreciate that it reports on a study of behavioral interventions such as those mentioned above: Specifically, discordant couples [couples where one partners is HIV positive and the other is not infected] were strongly counseled to use condoms and practice safe sex. That we witnessed no HIV transmissions after the intervention documents the success of the interventions in preventing the sexual transmission of HIV. The sentence in the Abstract reflects this success – nothing more, nothing less. Any attempt to refer to this or other of our publications and studies to bolster the fallacy that HIV is not transmitted heterosexually or homosexually is a gross misrepresentation of the facts and a travesty of the research that I have been involved in for more than a decade. If safe sex practices are followed, and if there are no complicating factors such as those mentioned above, the risk of HIV transmission can be as low as our studies suggest. . .IF. But many people misunderstand probability: they think that if the chance of misfortune is one in six, that they can take five chances without the likelihood of injury. This "Russian Roulette" misapprehension is dangerous to themselves and to others. Furthermore, complicating factors are often not evident or obvious in a relationship, so their perceived absence should not be counted on as an excuse not to practice safe sex.[41]

Despite the epidemiological science to the contrary, Stuart Brody, a sexologist at the University of Paisley, also denies the prevalence of vaginal transmission of HIV and dissuades people from using condoms. Brody states that research on condoms for preventing heterosexual transmission of HIV is flawed and that there exists no clear evidence that condoms prevent heterosexual transmission of HIV. He also states that the benefits of condom use for homosexual men in terms of preventing HIV infection are also disputable. Brody amazingly claims that the sexually transmitted HIV epidemic is due to anal intercourse and not vaginal sex. How then are we to explain the heterosexual HIV epidemic when more than 90% of heterosexuals with HIV/ AIDS report never engaging in anal sex? According to Brody, it is simple – people just do not tell the truth about having anal sex. In an interview with the BBC in 2003, Brody said, "The combination of serious illegality and taboo makes it something that it is not likely to generate correct answers when researchers ask and is not likely to be the subject of public health interventions." Brody also states that high rates of anal gonorrhea infections in women offers proof of prevalent anal sex. However, a well-understood complication of vaginal infections, including gonorrhea, is their spread from the lower vagina to the upper anus, a fact that does not require advanced knowledge of female anatomy. Nevertheless, Brody concludes that in North America and Europe, heterosexuals who have HIV were infected from injection drug use, and those who did not inject drugs became infected during anal intercourse.

What about Africa, where nearly all HIV infections occur among heterosexuals and injection drug use is exceedingly rare? Brody states the following:

> Public health authorities have long believed that the preponderance of AIDS cases in Africa are attributable to 'heterosexual transmission'; most people silently assume this rubric to indicate penile–vaginal intercourse only. Recent epidemiologic analyses suggest that the majority of HIV cases in sub-Saharan Africa may be due to non-sterile health care practices. ...both homosexuality and heterosexual anal intercourse are more prevalent in Africa than has traditionally been believed. ...perhaps the majority of HIV transmission not accounted for by iatrogenic [medical instrument] exposure could be accounted for by unsuspected and unreported penile–anal intercourse.[42]

The notion that HIV spread rampantly in Africa through contaminated medical instruments stems from a theory of how AIDS originated in Africa in the first place. The theory states that African hunters had contact with Simian Immune Deficiency Virus (SIV), a virus very similar to HIV found in apes, and the virus mutated to infect humans. The theory goes on to say that bush hunters exposed to the virus spread it to others through reused vaccination syringes and other unsterile medical equipment. This idea has been the basis for David Gisselquist, an economics consultant, to state "For the last 15 years, the AIDS establishment somehow got on to the notion that we need to scare people about sex to prevent HIV transmission."[43]

In response to Gisselquist's proclamation that HIV has spread through Africa by non-sterile medical practices, the World Health Organization launched a multinational investigation. The results flat out refuted Gisselquist, finding "no compelling evidence that unsafe injections are a predominant mode of HIV-1 transmissions in sub-Saharan Africa."[44] The Human Sciences Research Council in South Africa also spent precious resources to debunk an offshoot of Gisslequist's notions. According to Gisselquist, cases in which HIV negative women have HIV positive children, and these cases do occur, must result from HIV transmission in African medical settings. This study too concluded that there was no evidence for widespread medical HIV transmission. HIV infected infants born to uninfected mothers were occurring when infant feeding practices inadvertently exposed children to receiving HIV-contaminated milk. Specifically, the virus can be transmitted when HIV positive women feed babies or pool their milk to feed babies other than their own. Nearly one-third of the breast milk destined for use with hospitalized breastfed children has evidence of HIV contaminated milk.

Michael Carey of Syracuse University and I debunked Brody's claims about vaginal intercourse and condoms in 1995, and our comments apply equally well to Brody and Gisselquist's claims today:

> Brody's arguments are not grounded in an objective review of the literature on HIV transmission. Selective and biased reviewing cannot override a decade of sound virology, epidemiology, and clinical research. Unfortunately, Brody's conclusions contribute more to public misconceptions and myth perpetuation than they do to the scientific literature. Interpretations such as these have the potential for grave outcomes, especially in times when AIDS conspiracy theories abound, heterosexually acquired HIV infections (in the United States) are on the increase and heterosexual transmission of HIV accounts for approximately 90% of infections in women and 60% of infections in men, worldwide. Brody's paper appears to be a throwback to a time when 'reticence and even disbelief in the existence of heterosexual transmission of HIV by many policy makers was an extraordinary phenomenon, expressive of our limitless ability to deny logic and evidence when we choose to.[45]

Cashing In

Most AIDS pseudoscientists argue against treating people with HIV medications because they believe that HIV does not cause AIDS. In some cases, it appears that the aims of the pseudoscientists are to make a name for themselves. Others seem to just enjoy being contrarians, gaining attention by swimming against the mainstream. It also seems that some pseudoscientists are simply trapped in a level of suspicion that filters evidence to arrive at their pre-conceived notions. Still others may be playing out some grudge against the scientific establishment. Indeed, some may just be misguided. In any of these cases, pseudoscientists are not evil. If anything, the sense of disrespect and professional isolation experienced by AIDS pseudoscientist is sad. But then there is one class of pseudoscientist that is malevolent, perhaps even evil. It is those who profit from quackery and exploit the psychologically vulnerable, such as people diagnosed with HIV infection who are in denial. Specifically, those pseudoscientists who dissuade people with HIV from taking medications that can help them only to sell untested remedies, vitamins, and potions cross the line between what could arguably be protected free speech and are perpetrating harm to the public health.

To cure AIDS, people in the United States have been injecting Aloe Vera. People in Mexico have been using Ozone Therapy. Hyperthemia induced by hot water baths have been used in Latvia. Pesticides in Zambia. I have known people with HIV who cannot afford food but purchase expensive potions from Africa and exotic berry juices from South America. People have stopped taking life-prolonging medications and started taking health threatening mega-doses of vitamins.

Perhaps the first quack AIDS curer was Dr. Hulda Clark, whose book The *Cure for all HIV and AIDS* is sold worldwide. I have seen this book on the shelves of every major bookstore chain from Seattle to Cape Town. In fact, it is often the only book on AIDS in the health section. Why would this book not be popular? Who does not want to cure AIDS? Especially when it is as easy as Clark says. According to her, you can be HIV negative in 6 weeks! She reports 53 case studies of AIDS completely cured. The inside of the book even has a warning not to delay:

> You may not have time to read this entire book if you are sick with AIDS. You may wish to skip the part about how HIV infection is caused and go directly to the HIV curing recipe.

What is the cure for AIDS that Dr. Clark is selling? Well, first you have to kill the flukes, the worm like parasites that migrate from the intestines to the thalamus gland and cause the disease. But the trick is to kill the flukes at all of the stages of their development. You will need extra strength black walnut hull tincture, wormwood capsules, and clove capsules. Note that family members are instructed to also take the walnut hull in order to avoid reinfecting the person after they are cured. And in case the person may have other infections, Clark gives detailed instructions on how to build a Zapper – an electrical device that kills just about any microbe one may be afflicted with.

Another notorious AIDS pseudoscientist who has cashed in is German vitamin entrepreneur Matthias Rath. He sells vitamins and micronutrients – which he claims, when they are taken in high quantities – will cure AIDS and Cancer. Supposedly at the core of Rath's opposition to HIV treatments is a conspiracy involving pharmaceutical companies, the US government, Bill Gates, Bill Clinton and various other promoters of HIV medications. As

I mentioned earlier, Rath claims there is a global conspiracy to commit genocide against Africa. He tries to convince people to stop taking "toxic" drugs that will kill them and to take his vitamins instead. Rath sells several vitamin remedies to bolster nearly every bodily system and treat numerous ailments. One of his remedies for the immune system is a product called Immunocell a "daily nutritional supplement" that contains a combination of "various essential nutrients in a synergistic composition that assists in the creation of new blood and therefore, reinforces the natural immune system of the body."[46] Rath's products are sold worldwide, not just in Africa.

What makes Rath an AIDS pseudoscientist and not just your garden-variety vitamin pusher is that he has conducted unethical experiments that he claims have shown vitamins reverse AIDS. Rath and David Rasnick have a brochure titled "Clinical Proof: Micronutrients Reverse the Course of AIDS!" in which they proclaim a "Scientific breakthrough in fighting HIV/AIDS – Naturally." In these dark examples of pseudoscience at its worst, people given mega-doses of vitamins without ethical over site. People died in these so-called studies. The acts were so egregious that the South African Treatment Action Campaign launched legal action against Rath and his associates.[47] In June 2008, the South African courts found Rath guilty and ruled the studies unlawful.

There are now countless natural cures for AIDS being peddled in Africa. One such potion is Ubehjane, which is sold throughout southern Africa as a traditional medicine. A truck driver named Zeblon Gwala claims he had a dream where his dead grandfather, who had been a traditional healer, gave him the recipe for Ubehjane, so he started making and selling the concoction of 89 herbs from seven different African countries. The South African government actually tested Ubehjane and found that it is not harmful, but no one has shown that it works. Herbal remedies are springing up in ancestral dreams throughout Africa, and one herbal remedy in South Africa sells for as much as $200 a treatment. A non-natural cure for AIDS – a product called Tetrasil – has also spread in Zambia. People living with HIV/AIDS in Zambia were reportedly abandoning their antiretroviral drugs for Tetrasil and other ineffective remedies promoted as cures. After investigating, the Zambian government found that Tetrasil is a pesticide used in swimming pools and ultimately banned its use. The President of Gambia Yahya Jammeh claims to have discovered the cure for AIDS and asthma and actively treats patients himself. However, the contents of the cure are unknown, but the results are that it has not cured anyone of AIDS but has skyrocketed President Jammeh's popularity. At the root, so to speak, of much of the proliferation of quack cures in South Africa has resulted from the former Health Minister herself blocking the use of HIV treatments and suggesting nutritional remedies instead, particularly beetroot, lemon, garlic, and African potatoes. The problem has become so widespread that the government of Malawi has drafted a law to prevent traditional healers from claiming that they can cure HIV/AIDS and religious leaders from advising that people give up treatment for prayer.

Another nutritionist cashing in on HIV/AIDS is Gary Null, who sells vitamins, nutritional remedies, air filtration devices, magnetic products, books, DVDs, pet care products, super foods, anti-aging tablets, hair products, kosher foods, and much more. Gary Null has had his own radio talk show and he has even produced movies on the conspiracy behind AIDS, such as *AIDS Inc.* and *AIDS: A second opinion.* In his book *AIDS: A Second Opinion*, Null seems to repeat what other denialists have claimed. He states that the cure for AIDS is available, but the pharmaceutical industry is suppressing it. Null is described by the Internet watchdog group Quackwatch.com in this way:

> Null is prone to see conspiracies behind many of the things he is concerned about. One of his targets has been the pharmaceutical industry, which, he says, "cannot afford to have an alternative therapy accepted." He promotes hundreds of ideas that are inaccurate, unscientific, and/or unproven. He calls fluoridation "deadly" and has spoken out against immunization, food irradiation, amalgam fillings, and many forms of proven medical treatment. His series on "The Politics of Cancer," which was published in *Penthouse* magazine in 1979 and 1980, promoted unproven methods that he said were being "suppressed" by the medical establishment. His lengthy series, "Medical Genocide," began appearing in *Penthouse* in 1985 with an article calling our medical care system a "prescription for disaster" and claiming that modern medicine has had virtually no effect on heart disease, cancer, and arthritis. Other articles in the series promoted chiropractic and homeopathy, claimed that effective nutritional methods for treating AIDS were being suppressed, claimed that chelation therapy was safe and effective for treating heart disease, and endorsed several treatments for cancer that the American Cancer Society recommends against. His Web site contains a huge amount of misinformation and bad advice.[48]

Countless lesser known, although not necessarily less dangerous, entrepreneurs also sell AIDS cures. It is Null, Clark, Rath, Rasnick, and Giraldo, who deserve the most severe attention because the balance between protecting free speech and protecting the public health is so obviously breached.

AIDS pseudoscience fuels denialism and builds a market for quackery, first by convincing people to doubt medical science and second by claiming that HIV treatments are toxic poison. Convincing people that their failing immune system is their own fault because of their lifestyle or drug use creates a vulnerability. Once established, the vulnerability causes people to reach out for help, which is offered in the form of natural remedies and cures. Even among those who may not abandon their HIV medications completely, vitamin pushers and entrepreneurs will sell products to anyone who buys them.

Beyond the potential harm of the products themselves, taking money from the poor for bogus treatments is beyond criminal. Unlike the Loch Ness Monster and your friendly alien abductor, vitamin pushers and AIDS quacks play a truly lethal role in denialism. How people become lured to denialism is typically not through direct exposure to AIDS pseudoscience, but rather, it is denialist journalism and the mystique of the AIDS conspiracy.

Denialist Journalism and Conspiracy Theories

Today's scientists are almost wholly dependent upon the goodwill of government researchers and powerful peer-review boards, who control a financial network binding together the National Institutes of Health, academia, and the biotech and pharmaceutical industries. Many scientists live in fear of losing their funding. "Nobody is safe," one NIH-funded researcher told me. "The scientific-medical complex is a $2 trillion industry," says former drug developer Dr. David Rasnick, who now works on [Dr. Rath's] nutrition-based AIDS programs in Pretoria, South Africa. "You can buy a tremendous amount of consensus for that kind of money."

Celia Farber, Harper's Magazine, 2006

How is it that seemingly intelligent and often well-educated people can come to believe that HIV does not cause AIDS? Why is pseudoscience accepted over sound science? Journalists, mathematicians, chemists, physicists, lawyers, and nearly anyone who starts a web site seems capable of countering 25 years of biomedical research. Their message is one that anyone would surely welcome; that HIV is harmless. They also say that AIDS is only a problem for the most marginalized people and it is of their own doing. The journalists who propagate denialism hold the most appeal to those who mistrust science, medicine and government; the new anti-establishment truth seekers who look toward the Internet for their sense of reality. Denialists share much in common with 9/11 Truth groups and those who doubt that man ever landed on the moon. All conspiracy theories link a corrupt government with big business to hoax the American public. Whether the focus be on the Defense Department in cahoots with the oil industry, NASA working with aerospace contractors, or the NIH in the service of Big Pharma, the motivation for staging the 9/11 terrorist attacks, faking a lunar landing, and creating the AIDS virus is the same; money. Take these excerpts from various web sites for example:

But, in order to unleash their foreign/military campaigns without taking all sorts of flak from the traditional wing of the conservative GOP – which was more isolationist, more opposed to expanding the role of the federal government, more opposed to military adventurism abroad – they needed a context that would permit them free rein. The events of 9/11 rode to their rescue.... a catastrophic and catalyzing event – like a new Pearl Harbor.[1]

NASA raised approximately 30 billion dollars pretending to go to the moon. This could have been used to pay off a large number of people, providing significant motivation for complicity. In variations of this theory, the space industry is characterized as a political economy, much like the military industrial complex, creating fertile ground for its own survival.[2]

Who profits from mandatory testing for pregnant women? That's a whole new market for the tests opened up right there. Who profits from government mandates on drug therapies? Who will benefit from mandatory vaccines? We don't have it yet, but we're getting real close. This is no conspiracy. It's just business. We recognize it when corporations and governments do this in other areas of our lives. I'm always surprised at how so few critical thinkers, social leaders and liberal progressives recognize it in AIDS.[3]

The AIDS pseudoscientists discussed in the previous chapter would have remained in obscurity if not for a small group of journalists who have picked up their cause and sensationalized their writings. There are several examples of newspapers and tabloids promoting AIDS conspiracy theories and denialism. In 2007, for example, cancer specialist and Professor Karol Sikora published the article "The AIDS epidemic that never was and why political correctness influences too much medical spending" in the UK daily Mail. Atieno Amisi wrote the story "Raising dissenting voices on HIV link to AIDS" published in Business Daily Africa about the enlightenment offered by Christine Maggiore's experiences and the myth that HIV causes AIDS. Countless other newspapers have picked up the mystery and intrigue offered by a good conspiracy story.

Freelance denialist journalists have also managed to work their way into mainstream media. In one case in particular, Celia Farber has managed to get denialism into high profile popular media outlets. In most instances, Farber has exploited her connections to the publishing empire of her long time boyfriend Bob Guccione, including *Spin* and *Discover* magazines. Farber has also, however, been featured in *Harper's* magazine, bringing denialism to a height it would never have achieved otherwise. Less successful, though no less destructive, denialist journalists reach millions of readers via the Internet, particularly on the blogosphere. Denialist journalists, whether in print or in electronic publishing, use several classic techniques of propaganda and rhetoric to convince their readers that HIV does not cause AIDS. As we have already seen in AIDS pseudoscience, the underlying conspiracy behind AIDS is also not lost on freelance denialist journalists. Here I examine the rhetorical tools of denialism including the use of AIDS conspiracies.

A Web of Denialism

Denialism flourishes on the Internet. The Internet has done for denialism in the new millennium what transcontinental air travel did for the spread of HIV itself in the 1970s. In the 1990s, denialism emerged and spread throughout the world via the Internet. The Internet has made pseudoscience as accessible, or perhaps even more accessible, than quality medical science. However, the most easily accessed pseudoscience is delivered by denialist journalists who often write commentaries for various online magazines as well as maintain their own web sites. Even South African president Thabo Mbeki is said to have solidified his HIV/AIDS denialist views by accessing and ultimately buying into denialist web sites.

Denialist web sites use links to band together. In the world of denialism, links create an impression that there are thousands or tens of thousands of people who question the medical facts of AIDS. Internet users who enter a denialist web site are easily lost in what can seem like an endless loop of denialist propaganda and pseudoscience. Amidst "AIDS myths," "AIDS frauds," "Reappraising AIDS" and "Rethinking AIDS" there is an endless stream of pseudoscience and strange ideas, many discussed in the previous chapter. Conspiracy theories abound, implicating the US military, the National Institutes of Health, CDC, the CIA, Bill Gates, Bill Clinton, and Bono in a global plot to sell HIV treatments.

For people who innocently search the Internet for AIDS information, denialists are at best confusing and at worst convincing. Tragically, the people who are most vulnerable to denialism are those who have recently tested HIV positive and those who know someone who has tested HIV positive. Disinformation encountered online can bewilder anyone, and someone who is emotionally distraught can be easily pulled out to sea. Imagine that you or someone you care for has just tested HIV positive and you get online to find information about this new devastating diagnosis. Imagine that you search the Internet and come across the following:

> There is no cure for AIDS. There are drugs that can slow down the HIV virus and slow down the damage to your immune system. There is no way to "clear" HIV from the body. Other drugs can prevent or treat opportunistic infections (OIs). In most cases, these drugs work very well. The newer, stronger ARVs have also helped reduce the rates of most OIs. A few OIs, however, are still very difficult to treat.[4]

Then at the click of your mouse and you find this:

A growing group of bio-medical scientists claim the cause of AIDS is still unknown. These heretics do not believe in the lethal AIDS virus called HIV. They claim that the virus is indeed harmless. Most of them think AIDS is also not sexually trans-mitted; it probably has toxic causes. People die because they are poisoned to death by toxic antiviral drugs. Part of the AIDS dissidents even question the existence of a virus entity. These HIV skeptics say that the AIDS virus has never really been isolated, and the AIDS tests are worthless.[5]

Which web site would you want to believe? Where would you turn for more information? Who would you know to trust? It is easy to see how people can be lured into denialism. The same understandable preference for information that speaks of a cure is seen off the Internet. Nathan Geffen, an AIDS activist with the Treatment Action Campaign in South Africa, described to me essentially the same scenario for South Africans living with HIV/AIDS who may not even have Internet access. He told me that for the average poor person living in a South African township, the trip to their public health clinic is sheer hell, often arriving as early as 6 am only to sit in the stuffy over-crowded waiting room for 4–5 hours. Finally they get seen by an angry over-worked nurse for 5–10 minutes. They then must go and stand in the pharmacy queue for perhaps two hours. They get their medicine while the pharmacist barks unintelligible orders at them, sometime in a language they barely under-stand. If the person works as a laborer or sells goods in the informal sector, the insult is added to injury by having lost a day of earnings.

The alternative that Geffen describes is going to someone like Tine van der Maas, an infamous South African AIDS healer implicated in the deaths of people who come to her for traditional care. She is nice, gives people a cup of tea, sits and talks for half-hour, explaining that the HIV medicines are toxic. She then gives people a garlic concoction, which she says will cure AIDS/asthma/diabetes, whatever. It might cost a bit of money, but the person does not lose a day of work and they have a nice experience with someone from their own community who genuinely seems to care about them. The trans-mission of denialism is the same on and off the Internet when it comes to hooking in a vulnerable person to persuade them not to get tested for HIV or not to accept treatment.

The Internet does not distinguish between the wheat and chaff, and neither do most Internet users. In one study, Gretchen Berland and her colleagues found that higher quality health information online is frequently geared toward the well educated, with all English web sites in their study requiring high school reading levels or higher to merely comprehend the information. Their study showed that more than half of the health information found on the Internet is either incomplete or inaccurate. Research has also shown that people who have HIV/AIDS and use the Internet to learn about AIDS treatments find it difficult to distinguish credible medical information from even the most dubious false claims for an AIDS cure. In one study conducted by my research group, AIDS patients viewed a web site declaring a cure for AIDS concocted from a solution of goat's blood serum nearly as credibly as HIV treatment information from the American Medical Association.

The Internet offers limitless opportunities for disinformation. The sheer volume of bogus HIV treatment information found online is mind boggling. A simple Google search for AIDS cures will get you "66 reasons to think twice about the HIV test" at Christine Maggiore's Alive & Well AIDS Alternatives, "Do antibody tests prove HIV infection" by Valendar F. Turner and Huw Christie, "Influenza vaccination and false positive HIV results" by Christian P. Erickson, "Everybody reacts positive on the ELISA test for HIV" by Roberto Giraldo, "Viral load and the PCR : Why they can't be used to prove HIV infection" by Christine Johnson, and "Viral load of crap" by Paul Philpott and Christine Johnson.

Unlike mainstream media, there is no editorial oversight and no accountability on the Internet. The Internet truly is the Wild West where anything goes. The Internet does not get any more free-ranging than in the blogosphere.

Blah-Blah-Bloggers

Within the web of denialism, there are numerous email list-serves and blogs, ranting places for those with apparently lots of time on their hands. Blogs can be an effective medium for stirring up controversy and gaining attention. The best-known blog in denialism is Liam Scheff's "Liam's World" {http://liamscheff.com/blog/}. Here you will find Liam's articles on war, creationism, global warming, politics, and AIDS. Liam Scheff is most well known among denialists for calling attention to HIV positive orphaned children who were enrolled in clinical trials for antiretroviral therapies in New York City. Scheff's Internet postings included a story he wrote for *Hustler* magazine titled *Guinea Pig Kids*. Ultimately, the BBC picked up the story and produced a documentary of the same title, only to later publicly retract and apologize. The entire drama, from Liam's initial postings, to the triumph of the mainstream coverage, to the humiliation of BBC's apology, played out on Liam's Blog. The blogosphere has added a new dimension to denialism. Bizarre ideas have a way of feeding off each other, often escalating to new heights. That is precisely what we see when reading through these blogs. Denialists often make their voices heard on the mainstream science and health blogs. There are instances when denialist blogging has gotten out of control and blogs have been shut down because of denialist takeovers. For example, it has been the case, more than once, that denialists and anti-denialists have entered a blog creating an endless loop of character assassinations and personal attacks.

The Great AIDS Debate?

Denialist journalists insistently demand for an open and fair debate on whether HIV causes AIDS. Once there was a need for legitimate debate on the cause of AIDS. In 1981 before the cause of AIDS was established, there was good reason to debate whether a virus was the cause of AIDS. There was also considerable debate about the modes of HIV transmission. In the 1980s, most scientists agreed that HIV is spread through sexual contact, sharing injection drug equipment, and exposure to HIV contaminated blood. But there were dissident scientists who questioned whether HIV was transmitted by insect bites. Some experts believed that insects transmitted HIV, particularly mosquitoes in a manner similar to malaria. Belle Glade Florida is one migrant farming community that received particular attention in this debate because this town, which sits on the edge of Lake Okeechobee, is ravaged by mosquitoes and had a rapidly growing HIV epidemic. Anyone who has driven through Belle Glade knows the abundance of mosquitoes there and knows that any disease that is spread by mosquitoes would be a disaster for Belle Glade. The legitimate debate about whether HIV was spread by mosquitoes played out in conferences and the most prestigious scientific journals. Ultimately, dissident scientists conducted research in Belle Glade, showing that in fact HIV infection was least common in babies and the elderly, the very same people with the most mosquito bites. The debate on mosquitoes spreading HIV ended with dissident scientists accepting the data and moving on.

The evidence that HIV causes AIDS is as compelling as the evidence that the virus is not transmitted by mosquitoes. Nonetheless, the outcry for a debate about whether HIV causes AIDS remains a fixation of denialists. Denialists claim that there urgently needs to be a debate between the "foremost establishment scientists and the best-credentialed dissenting ones." Of course, they claim that AIDS scientists continually refuse to participate in a debate with any "dissident" out of fear of being shown wrong.[6]

From the denialists' perspective, AIDS scientists are afraid to debate HIV causing AIDS because they risk exposure of the truth. Charles Geshekter, prominent denialist who was on South African President Mbeki's AIDS panel, states that it serves no advantage to AIDS scientists to participate in an open debate on the cause of AIDS:

From what I would consider to be the inherent flaws and weaknesses in the HIV=AIDS infectious theory, I think what would happen would be that the public would see that the emperor has no clothes. And I think that you would see that the notion that the HIV infectious viral theory as science would be exposed for the ideology that it really has become. I don't think it could withstand a close, careful questioning. Further evidence of that is the way that those of us who are dissidents have had our views censored or not given a public forum to express those views. And so, if I were in the (Robert) Gallo (David) Ho camp, the last thing I would want would be an open, unfettered, robust exchange of scientific ideas.[7]

From the perspective of AIDS scientists, the question as to whether HIV causes AIDS is settled. Debating HIV as the cause of AIDS would itself legitimize the very question, as it did in South Africa when the President invited just such a debate on his Advisory Panel. Because denialism relies on half-truths and misrepresentations, it is easy to get caught in their tangled argument. The anti-denialist web site aidstruth.org lists four reasons why scientists should not be drawn into a debate about the cause of AIDS with denialists. These include (1) the debate has simply been settled: HIV causes AIDS, AIDS kills, and AIDS can be treated with significant success by the use of antiretroviral therapy; (2) the information proving that HIV causes AIDS is already in the peer-reviewed science literature. Denialists ignore, misunderstand or willfully misrepresent the known facts. Although scientists should not debate denialists, it is the role of scientists to enlighten denialists in order to help them better understand the available information; (3) debating denialists dignifies their position. AIDS scientists hold that the best way for dissidents to persuasively communicate their views is by publishing in the peer-reviewed scientific literature; and (4) scientists believe that their time is better spent conducting research into HIV/AIDS and/or educating the public about the facts about this virus and the deadly disease it causes.[8]

Unable to engage AIDS scientists in a debate about the cause of AIDS, denialists have been left to deconstruct AIDS on their own.

Deconstructing AIDS

Denialists who deconstruct HIV as the cause of AIDS remind me of when my brother-in-law tried to fix the engine of his 1968 Chevy. He took the whole car apart on his front lawn, rebuilt the engine, and had several nuts and bolts left laying there. HIV/AIDS deconstructionists face the same fate. Stemming from a basic distrust of science, deconstruction implies AIDS was "constructed" in the first place, relating back to Peter Duesberg's premise that the AIDS virus was invented. As Christine Maggiore has articulated her basis for deconstructing AIDS:

My skepticism came out of concern and compelled me to dig deeper, go beyond unquestioning acceptance. When I looked closer and applied some critical think-ing, I found the primary assumptions about AIDS just don't add up. There's a great deal of information portrayed as true and certain that is far from absolute or clearly established, disturbing omissions of inconvenient facts, lots of poorly conceived and constructed studies, biased research, and some fairly overt manipulation of statistics.[9]

Biologists and medical scientists universally accept that HIV infection is the most complex viral disease encountered in human history. As an RNA virus as opposed to a DNA virus, HIV replicates in the reverse sequence of other viruses and then integrates itself with the DNA of immune system cells. For denialist deconstructionists, not understanding the basic biology and pathology of HIV and failing to see the logic in how HIV causes AIDS is the basis for their doubt. However, misunderstanding AIDS is insufficient and does not lead to denialism. Rather, people get hooked into denialism by becoming lost in a sea of rhetoric and propaganda. Proliferated mostly by a small group of freelance journalists, denialism can be quite persuasive to anyone who does not understand the basic science of AIDS. I now turn to the rhetorical techniques most commonly found in denialist journalism.

Denialist Journalism Meets AIDS Pseudoscience

The world of denialism revolves around its journalists, particularly those with web sites. Denialist journalists include the whole spectrum, from widely known columnists such as Tom Bethell, to freelancers such as Celia Farber and David Crowe, to journalist wannabes and bloggers. Their subject matter is drawn from the lives of denialist activists and the writings of AIDS pseudoscientists. Table 4.1 shows some of the milestones in journalism propagating denialism. Denialist journalism is well recognized for using a gamut of rhetorical tools that allow them to misrepresent pseudoscience as science. In the absence of editorial oversight, the possibilities seem endless.

Morphing Science and Technobabble

Morphing science simply transforms basic facts into disinformation. One strategy for morphing science involves selecting a bunch of disconnected statements from legitimate sources and pasting them into a text meant to sound scientific although almost always impossible to follow. Even scientifi-cally trained readers will get lost in the illogic of morphed science. Morphed science can convince the untrained reader that the author is knowledgeable about AIDS while not understanding a word of what they are saying. And that is of course the point.

Table 4.1 Examples of journalism propagating HIV/AIDS denialism

Publication	Impact
Jeanne Lenzer, Peter's Principle, *Discover* magazine, June, 2008. This featured article tells Duesberg's story, again. Highlights his new old ideas on cancer and his hope for vindication.	*Discover* magazine is widely read and available on news stands everywhere. The exposure to Duesberg as he was slipping into obscurity brought him new attention.
Karol Sikora, The Aids epidemic that never was and why political correctness influences too much medical spending, November, 21, 2007, the daily Mail (UK). Reports on adjusted AIDS surveillance projections that were reduced to more accurate levels.	Misconstrues the adjusted epidemiology to suggest that AIDS is not devastating populations and has unjustifiably pulled resources from other diseases, such as cancer.
Susan Kruglinski, Questioning the HIV Hive Mind? An interview with Celia Farber, long-serving chronicler of HIV dissidents, *Discover* magazine, October, 2006.	Interview with Celia Farber following the publication of her collection of magazine articles. The interview brought forward the growth of denialism over the years that Farber had been chronicling the "AIDS dissidents."
Celia Farber, "Out of Control," *Harper's* magazine, March 2006. Featured story on the continued censorship of Peter Duesberg and the unanswered questions about AIDS.	Considered to have a significant impact because of its visibility. AIDS scientists identified 50 significant errors and misrepresentations in the article.
Jamie Doran, BBC, "Guinea Pig Kids," 2005. Film that reported on orphaned children in New York taking part in NIH HIV treatment trials. Also picked up by Larry Flynt's *Hustler* magazine.	Instigated by Liam Scheff, the story ultimately resulted in children being removed from HIV treatment. The BBC came to learn they have been led astray by Scheff and apologized for producing the documentary.
Tom Bethell, "Inventing the AIDS Epidemic," Capitol Ideas Column, American *Spectator Magazine*, April 2000. Raises skepticism about the government, suggesting that the traditional diseases of Africa have become construed as AIDS.	This mainstream conservative magazine gave attention to denialism, drawing in a whole new and sympathetic audience.
Tom Bethell, "Could Duesberg be Right?," *National Review*, August, 1992. Discusses misconstrued events reported in mainstream media to raise questions about whether Duesberg will ultimately be shown right on AIDS.	As a well recognized conservative commentator, Bethell has brought denialism to a new readers who probably had never before heard of Duesberg and his ideas. In this article, Bethell discuss the idea of HIV testing in army recruits as not lining up with AIDS cases, an idea later used by Henry Bauer.

South African attorney and self-taught AIDS expert Anthony Brink is notorious for patching together pieces of science to form a convoluted and inaccurate science-sounding argument. The following example refutes the known disease causing pathways of HIV. Note the final sentence, in which he mocks the urgency of AIDS:

Let's close our eyes and pretend just for now that reverse transcriptase has unambiguously been shown to exist as a distinct enzyme unique to retroviruses and not also a component of uninfected human cells, and that retroviruses exist outside textbooks, like Coffin's, and children's imaginations, as in the Superman cartoon movie *Cold Vengeance*: "a Roscoe's retrovirus...100 per cent fatal," and that retroviruses can be malevolent and have sufficient genetic complexity for the execution of their nefarious intentions, and that HIV is one of them. Killing off our CD4 immune cells. No evidence for that? OK, not attacking them directly, but hypnotizing them into committing suicide. Even those they haven't been anywhere near. Like telepathically. They call it "programmed cell-death." For 'AIDS sufferers' with sky-high CD4 cell counts, we'll think up an explanation another day. Likewise one for folks in peak health with cell counts at rock bottom. Who should be gasping in hospices. Overcome by opportunistic infections. Except that we're talking about some US Olympic athletes. HIV sits dormant in our cells, a lurking lentivirus, poised to jump out and attack us after about a decade or so. No, no, we've dumped that theory; the new one is that it replicates from the start, incredibly rapidly but being neutralised by antibodies, although not quite efficiently enough to avoid being eventually overrun. Actually that model is now in the toilet too, so we 'AIDS experts' are not too sure what to say anymore, but who wants to get bogged down by details when we've got to get out there and save lives? I mean let's keep our eye on the bigger picture. Because like hey, people are dying.[10]

The aim of morphing science is to sound scientific to the point of incomprehension. The same objective is also met by using technobabble; the use of jargon, buzzwords and highly esoteric language to give an impression of plausibility through mystification, misdirection, and obfuscation.[11] Technobabble should not be confused with jargon itself which is the peculiar language of a technical field, but is rather the use of jargon for the sake of persuasion. The objective of technobabble in denialism is to present a façade of science within which it is easy to lose track of the details. Like morphing science, the goal is that readers render the material credible even if utterly unintelligible. Matt Irwin, a denialist blogger offers the following example of technobabble:

The number of viruses estimated by viral load tests are based on measurements of RNA fragments, so that any change in overall RNA levels in the blood could potentially alter a person's viral load, even if this RNA does not come from HIV. Many antiretroviral drugs have a short-term antimicrobial effect, which can result in a temporary improvement in health, and they do this by directly inhibiting RNA and DNA synthesis. These drugs also cause reduced RNA and DNA synthesis in a wide variety of human cells including red blood cells, white blood cells, nerve cells, bone building cells, and muscle cells, which result in some of their most common adverse effects as reported in clinical trials. Microbes that have been found to be suppressed by these drugs include Pneumocystis carinii, Candida albicans, Enterobacter, Shigella, Salmonella, Klebsiella, Citrobacter, and E-coli, and many other microbes that have not yet been studied may also be affected.[12]

Portraying Science as Religion

There are countless religious overtones to denialism particularly the use of spiritual images to describe mainstream AIDS science. AIDS science is called an "orthodoxy" that is promoting "HIV equals AIDS dogma" and scientists who question whether HIV causes AIDS are said to be "excommunicated." South African President Thabo Mbeki stated, "In an earlier period in human history, these [dissidents] would be heretics that would be burnt at the stake!"[13] The tactic of redefining science as religion aims to reduce scientific evidence to faith. AIDS scientists are typically portrayed as evil doers or even Nazis pitted again truth seekers; such as the evil government scientist Robert Gallo pitted against the martyred researcher Peter Duesberg. The following examples illustrate how denialists use religious phrasing in describing AIDS science.

- The followers of the HIV=AIDS "religion" have no evidence that HIV exists, and even less that such a virus could lead to the collapse of the human immune system. But they want to silence anyone who doesn't follow their beliefs. Apparently, the publication of books questioning their faith is the next evil item on their hit list.[14]
- The claims for exclusive authority of "scientific peers" are no more valid than those of their legal counterparts nor those of their predecessors who wrote prescriptions in Latin, or those of their theological counterparts who determine what's moral or ethical via special connections with God.[15]

Canadian journalist David Crowe has even created a satirical prayer that he calls the AIDS Creed. Crowe says that science orthodoxy is revered by those who "believe" HIV causes AIDS and they should have their own prayer, which includes the following excerpt:

I believe that on the first day Robert Gallo created antibody tests. On the second day they separated the godly from the evil. On the third day those with the mark descended into the hell of AIDS and will not rise again until dead. Gallo, on the other hand, will ascend into heaven where he will be forgiven all his sins. He will be seated where he cannot reach the wallet of the Father Almighty. On the fourth day AZT was invented. On the fifth day it created its first miracle. On the sixth day people started dying.,. but it wasn't by AZT, all the faithful know it was HIV. On the seventh day it was discovered that HIV is heterosexually as well as homosexually transmitted – gay in America and straight in Africa. Because we, the priesthood, know that only gay men and Africans are sinners.[16]

Cherry Picking

This technique is a favorite of denialists. Cherry picking involves selecting a lone scientific finding and presenting it out of context to suit one's argument. The misuse of Nancy Padian's research findings on heterosexual transmission of HIV discussed in Chapter 3 exemplifies the denialist use of cherry picking. Rebecca Culshaw and Peter Duesberg both used cherry picking to draw erroneous conclusions about the findings from Rodriguez and colleagues 2006 study that reported initial viral load did not predict the rate of decline of CD4/T-Helper cells, also discussed in Chapter 3. In a remarkable twist, Culshaw further misuses the cherry picked result to propose an alternate model of AIDS caused by oxidization in the immune system. She published her untested theory in a journal that has served as a common outlet for denialist literature.

The Single Study Fallacy

No one scientific study ever "proves" anything. Scientists are cautious in drawing conclusions from even a series of experiments. Science requires that independent studies replicate a finding before it is taken as fact. Even then, there is hesitation to accept replicated research findings as "proof." To establish that HIV causes AIDS required countless laboratory, clinical, and epidemiological studies, all converging to a definitive conclusion. There is, of course, no single scientific paper proving that HIV causes AIDS. Rather, there are tens of thousands of papers containing a wide-range of evidence that, taken together, makes the overwhelmingly case that HIV causes immune system decline that ultimately results in AIDS. One could similarly ask to see the single physics experiment that proves a rocket can fly to the moon. There is no such experiment. Does that mean that a rocket cannot fly to the moon? The proof that a rocket can fly to the moon comes from thousands of experiments in physics as well as lunar flight itself. Is there a single study that proves that excessive exposure to the sun causes sun cancer? Or smoking causes lung cancer? Demanding a single study to prove HIV causes AIDS follows the same illogic.

Denialists state that because there is no one study that has proven HIV causes AIDS the science of AIDS is a fraud. As stated by Peter Duesberg, "There is not a single controlled epidemiological study to confirm the postulated viral etiology of AIDS."[17] Denialist Toby Getttins similarly states that

"There is NO SUCH THING as the HIV virus. If there was, don't you think that the multi-billion dollar AIDS industry would have produced a sample of it by now? Something that actually replicates in human tissue? But hey, prove me wrong: Cite the scientific papers showing isolation and replication of the virus."[18]

Another form of the single study fallacy involves selecting a single research article and using it as a source of proof. This version of the single study fallacy is the entire basis for Henry Bauer's analysis of HIV testing data to prove that HIV cannot cause AIDS. He uses a single study of HIV testing with US military recruits to predict AIDS cases ten years later. The single study analyzed HIV test results from over 1.1 million teenage applicants for US military service between the years 1985 and 1989. As described in Chapter 3, the study offered a glimpse of the HIV prevalence of youth enrolling in the military from across the United States during the first years of AIDS. Bauer incorrectly uses this single study as if it were representative of the populations most affected by AIDS. He misuses the study to claim that HIV cannot cause AIDS because the youth represented in the HIV positive tests do not reflect the people who have AIDS. Baurer commits the obvious error of treating data taken at different times from different people as if they were the same people observed over the years.

The most repugnant examples of single study fallacies are, however, those that actually execute bogus research to claim proof that HIV does not cause AIDS or that HIV treatments are poison. In the case of Matthias Rath and David Rasnick, South Africans living with HIV/AIDS avoided taking antiretroviral medications to take mega-doses of Dr. Rath's vitamins. The results of their dubious study of 15 people are used to claim proof that vitamins can reverse the course of AIDS.

Stuck in the 1980s

Denialist journalists rely heavily on research citations from the 1980s, a time when far less about AIDS was known. Part of the reason for reliance on old information may simply be that old studies are just as easily accessed on the Internet as new information. There is also frequent recycling of cited research among denialists. Even then, studies from the 1980s are manipulated to counter such basic facts as HIV causing AIDS and HIV transmission via vaginal intercourse. Falling back on research from the 80s allows denialists to recycle outdated research over what is now decades. Among the most notorious examples of misrepresenting AIDS research from the 1980s as current work comes from Celia Farber's 2006 book *Serious Adverse Events: An Uncensored History of AIDS*. Farber's book is marketed as "what the AIDS dissident scientists have to say today," but the book is stuck in the

80s with the only recent content coming from Farber's 2006 *Harper's* magazine article. Farber's book is really an anthology of her magazine articles published in the 1980s and 1990s.

Denialists also look back to the 1980s for failed predictions made then by AIDS scientists. Most notably the United States Health and Human Services Secretary at the time predicted in the famous 1984 press conference with AIDS scientist Robert Gallo that there would be a vaccine for HIV forthcoming in two years and a cure soon after. There were also predictions in 1987 that HIV would spread into the heterosexual population of the United States, although no one ever predicted that HIV would be spread randomly through the population. There were also unfulfilled predictions in the late 1980s about the course of AIDS and the development of treatments. The tactic of pointing back to unfulfilled predictions allows denialists to raise questions such as "If HIV really causes AIDS then why are all of these predictions wrong?" Obviously, in the 1980s we knew little about HIV and how it causes AIDS. In hindsight, predictions for how HIV epidemics have expanded have also been off-base because the mathematical models used to forecast the epidemic have been unable to account for the numerous factors that facilitate the spread of HIV.

Pushing Back the Goal Posts

Another common tactic of denialists is to demand even more specific evidence only to change the demand once the evidence is produced. Scientists Tara Smith and Steven Novella have described how denialists use pushing back the goal posts in their rhetoric:

> The strategy behind goalpost-moving is simple: always demand more evidence than can currently be provided. If the evidence is then provided at a later date, simply change the demand to require even more evidence, or refuse to accept the kind of evidence that is being offered. In the 1980s, HIV deniers argued that drug therapy for AIDS was ineffective, did not significantly prolong survival, and in fact was toxic and damaged the immune system. However, after the introduction of a cocktail of newer and more effective agents in the 1990s, survival rates did impressively increase. HIV deniers no longer accept this criterion as evidence for drug effectiveness, and therefore the HIV theory of AIDS. Even stacks of papers and books published on the subject are not enough.[19]

The claim that HIV has never been "purified" is another example of pushing back the goal posts because the demand changes as research advances. The Perth Group and Neville Hodgkinson, for example, stated that HIV tests were invalid because the virus had not been isolated. After evidence that HIV had been isolated, the demand changed such that the isolated virus was said to be "impure." Denialists now demand that the virus be isolated in "pure form," not contaminated by proteins from cells. As recently as 2008, David Crowe has stated that the virus has never been purified and that HIV tests are therefore invalid. The demand for a pure virus devoid of cellular proteins is impossible to meet as it defies the biological nature of virus replication. The pure virus myth is the latest spot to which the denialists have moved the goal posts in their efforts to invalidate HIV antibody testing.

Preying on Fears

Denialists exploit the reasonable fears that most anyone will have to a life threatening disease. This tactic is particularly destructive because it exploits people who may be most vulnerable to medical disinformation. Denialist and Texas math teacher Rebecca Culshaw, for example, tries to scare people away from HIV testing by stringing together nearly every falsehood anyone has ever uttered about testing HIV positive:

> Aside from the fact that many people who are perfectly healthy will be coerced into undergoing a regimen of medication that will inevitably cause long-term toxic effects (and often death), a more sinister complication is the violation of human rights that occurs following a positive HIV test. Every state in the United States and every province in Canada maintain a list of 'HIV carriers' in that region. Once diagnosed HIV positive, medical and life insurance can be denied, some carriers may be terminated, but worst of all, a death sentence is given and, contrary to every other disease known to man, even cancers that generally 100 percent fatal, hope is not allowed. Women are encouraged to abort their babies, and if they choose to carry their pregnancy to term, in many states they are forced to take antiretroviral drugs, and those drugs are forced on their babies as well. The babies themselves must be born Caesarean section, and in many states the highly beneficial practice of breast feeding is illegal.[20]

The Spin Machine

The very nature of denialism encompasses the manipulation of facts to suit a specific agenda, which is the definition of spin. Denialist spin occurs most often when an AIDS news event or change in policy is twisted in support of denialist claims. For example, news that an HIV vaccine is shown not to offer protection against the virus is spun by denialists as evidence that AIDS is not caused by an infectious agent. Similarly, the news that the Director of the United Nations AIDS program (UNAIDS) Dr. Peter Piot had announced that he would be stepping down from his post of more than decade at the end of his term was spun as a collapse of the UNAIDS. For example, Internet blogger Liam Scheff boasted that UNAIDS is "being taken apart and falling apart," as the head "doom-and-gloom sex-and-death cheerleader" Peter Piot resigned. Similar spin occurs each time the CDC or the World Health Organization adjusts its epidemiology statistics to reflect new sources of information or more accurate data. Denialists spin these updates as if the numbers were originally fabricated to exaggerate the AIDS problem. Spin aims to fit emerging facts into the preconceived beliefs held by denialists. Spin is also the favorite instrument of conspiracy theories, which themselves are at the root of denialist journalism.

AIDS Conspiracies and Denialism

It is easy to think that people who espouse conspiracy theories cannot possibly be serious. Rest assured they are quite serious, and surprisingly common. Like conspiracy theories in general, AIDS conspiracies help to organize what must seem like a chaotic and unexplainable set of circumstances. Just as religion brings meaning to the world, conspiracy theories explain the unexplainable. Denialism is entrenched in conspiracy thinking because conspiracies have explanatory value. Great powers such as government, industry, medicine, and science offer easy answers to the great complexities in life that are beyond our control. The conspiracy theory may seem wacky at first, but buying into a conspiracy theory brings order and meaning to even the most horrific catastrophes such as the holocaust, 9/11 terrorist attacks, and AIDS.

There are instances when people are proponents of multiple conspiracy theories. For example, Lynn Margulis is a Distinguished University Professor in the Department of Geosciences at University of Massachusetts and, like Peter Duesberg, she is a member of the National Academy of Sciences. Margulis is also a noted denialist who believes that the 9/11 terror attacks were part of a US government conspiracy against countries in the Middle East. She has said:

The 9/11 tragedy is the most successful and most perverse publicity stunt in the history of public relations. . . .Whoever is responsible for bringing to grisly fruition this new false-flag operation, which has been used to justify the wars in Afghanistan and Iraq as well as unprecedented assaults on research, education, and civil liberties, must be perversely proud of their efficient handiwork. Certainly, 19 young Arab men and a man in a cave 7,000 miles away, no matter the level of their anger, could not have masterminded and carried out 9/11: the most effective television commercial in the history of Western civilization. I suggest that those of us aware and concerned demand that the glaringly erroneous official account of 9/11 be dismissed as a fraud and a new, thorough, and impartial investigation be undertaken.[21]

Conspiracy theories often grow out of a historical fact that becomes the seed for suspicion. In the United States, the most notorious historical fact in public health that gives rise to AIDS conspiracy theories comes from the Tuskegee Syphilis Study. In 1932, the US Public Health Service enrolled 600 African American men into a study to observe the natural history of syphilis.

A total of 399 of them had syphilis and 201 did not. The men were not told the reason for the study or its rationale and were not provided with informed consent. Originally planned for 6 months, the study went on for 40 years. When penicillin became the standard drug for treating syphilis in 1947, the men where not offered treatment. The Tuskegee study gives good reason for African Americans to distrust the public health enterprise. In South Africa, there are known accounts of secret biological weapons programs that were undertaken by the white minority Apartheid government. Dr. Wouter Basson oversaw South African Apartheid government programs that sought race-specific bacteria, mass sterilization, and fatal poisons for potential use against blacks, should they have gained too much power. These historical facts lead to understandable mistrust in government and public health entities. They also provide a kernel of truth for later day conspiracy theories.[22]

Social psychologist Laura Bogart at Harvard University has studied AIDS conspiracy theories in African American communities. In her research, she has found that two out of three African Americans believe that the US government is not telling the truth about AIDS and 16% believe that AIDS was created by the government to control the Black population. Conspiracy beliefs regarding HIV treatments are also common, with more than half of people believing that a cure for AIDS is available but is being withheld from the poor and 7% even agreeing that the medicines doctors prescribe to treat HIV are poison. Bogart has done additional research in the United States and in South Africa that has demonstrated similar results, suggesting wide scale beliefs that AIDS is an instrument of genocide.

AIDS Genocide Conspiracies

The first AIDS conspiracy theory seems to have originated with an East German biologist named Jakob Segal in 1986. He is credited, or blamed, as having first created a pamphlet that stated that AIDS was invented by the US army for genocidal use. The conspiracy was picked up by numerous others and proliferated widely. The conspiracy generally goes like this. The AIDS virus was invented by the National Cancer Institute, that would be Robert Gallo, and the World Health Organization in a secret laboratory at the US military labs in Ft. Detrick, Maryland. The virus was made by combining bovine (cow) leukemia virus and visna (sheep) virus. The resulting combination virus was then injected into human tissue cultures and the AIDS virus was born. It was then distributed throughout Africa, Haiti, Brazil, Southern Japan and Central America by the World Health Organization concealed in a free smallpox vaccination. The virus was also distributed in the United States within the 1978 Hepatitis B vaccination program, when gay men and injection drug users in New York and San Francisco were vaccinated.

Variations of the genocide conspiracy have been propagated by political extremists as well as unsuspecting celebrities. I recall when actor Will Smith was interviewed by Barbara Walters and he expressed his views about the AIDS plight in black America being instituted by the government. The most publicized of genocidal AIDS conspiracy theorists is Leonard Horowitz whose book *Emerging Viruses: AIDS & Ebola- Nature, Accident, or Intentional?* became a focal point in the 2008 US presidential campaign when Barack Obama's controversial pasture Rev. Jeremiah Wright cited the book as the basis for his comments that HIV was invented to kill blacks. Horowitz was also the guest speaker at a presidential campaign information forum held by Texas congressman Ron Paul's candidacy. Dr. Horowitz urged the presidential hopeful to be bold and take on the "petrochemical-pharmaceutical polluters and public health safety violators."

Another faction of the genocidal conspiracies promotes the idea that it is not AIDS itself but AIDS treatments that are part of a global attempt to kill Africans. The use of HIV treatments to commit genocide, however, is more akin to the Big Pharma genre of conspiracy theories.

Big Pharma Conspiracies

Pharmaceutical companies are, of course, in business for profit and there is plenty of history of Big Pharma engaging in exploitation and questionable practices. It is these historical realities that fuel the Big Pharma conspiracy, extending well beyond the drug companies themselves. Most Big Pharma-conspiracies tie together the US government, philanthropists, and anyone who tries to get antiretroviral treatments to people living with HIV/AIDS. These are the conspiracies that are most closely linked to the most ruthless denialists, those who sell fake treatments and cures. Some typical conspiracy theorizing in the denialist lore include the following:

- **Matthias Rath:** Against the will of the people of the world, who once set up the UN as an international body to improve the lives of all mankind, these drug-related interest groups abused these United Nation's bodies in a desperate attempt trying to block this breakthrough from reaching all mankind... The people and the governments of the world have to decide whether they are ready to stop being manipulated by the pharmaceutical industry and embrace instead the scientific knowledge that is now available to fight the global HIV/AIDS epidemic with effective, safe and affordable natural means.[23]
- **David Rasnick:** President Clinton did his bit to thicken the protective fog encasing the AIDS Blunder. Last summer he declared AIDS to be a risk to the national security of the United States. That action allowed at least three additional federal institutions to play a direct role in maintaining and

protecting the fiction of a global AIDS pandemic. These institutions are the Federal Bureau of Investigation (FBI), the Central Intelligence Agency (CIA), and the National Security Agency (NSA). The involvement of the FBI, CIA, and NSA in AIDS represents a far greater threat to our freedoms than to HIV.[24]

Of course, the Big Pharma conspiracy is much broader than just HIV/ AIDS. Journalist David Crowe, for example, has written extensively on the corruption of Big Pharma in promoting cancer treatment, claiming that cancer diagnostic tests and treatments, just like AIDS treatments, are poison for profit. Crowe advises us to be skeptical of the cancer industry's prevention-as-detection message. He warns that mammograms and prostate cancer screening are questionable in that they "raise the number of unnecessary interventions and, in the case of mammograms, may themselves contribute to cancer risk." Crowe says that neither mammograms nor prostate screening have been proven to reduce cancer mortality in a large population. His argument is that the medical care industry promotes screening and treatments based on "the power and prestige of the medical establishment," overlooking alternative and natural treatments which are safe and effective.[25] How is it possible that safer and effective treatments are not the scientific standard for AIDS and cancer treatment? Crowe says the answer is simple. There is widespread corruption in the peer review system that suppresses natural remedies in order to protect the interests of the pharmaceutical industry, the censorship conspiracy.

Censorship Conspiracies

Early in the lore of denialism the most common conspiracy concerned the alleged censorship of Peter Duesberg and his questioning HIV as the cause of AIDS. This conspiracy evolved into the broader conspiracy that says anyone who questions the cause of AIDS will experience censorship and ridicule. The view is that only a conspiracy of censorship can explain why Duesberg, Harvey Bialy, David Rasnick and other "great scientists" could not compete for NIH funding and publish their work in respectable scientific journals. Censorship against alternative views on AIDS explains why these scientists suffered such a fate. Denialists say they are victims of censorship under the threat of eviction from professional societies as well as threats to terminate their employment. Television and radio as well as the print media censor their views. Denialists believe that censorship has the direct effect of modifying behavior such that alternative views on AIDS are never voiced, leading to the logical conclusion that there are many more denialists out there than we can possibly know.

A fundamental element of the censorship conspiracy relies on the role of peer review in science as an instrument of suppressing new ideas. Earlier I discussed Duesberg and his associate David Rasnick's accounts of the peer review conspiracy. The peer review conspiracy asserts that scientists act on selfish interests by opposing new ideas to defend the status quo. Science is viewed as a cutthroat and backstabbing enterprise. According to denialists, the entire anonymous peer review system in science is corrupt and self-protecting. Denialists consider peer-review a clever smokescreen to give scientists control over research funding that promotes their own ideas – even when it is not their own research. The conspiracy extends to all peer-review, enabling a clique of scientists to control a much larger number of scientists, for their own benefit – financial and otherwise. Kelly Brennan-Jones, a psychologist at State University of New York in Brockport, reviewed Duesberg's book and supports the conclusion that there is a conspiracy to silence him. She wrote:

> Silence indeed equals death; silence about the true causes of AIDS, silence about the purported "cure" shoved down our throats and shoved down the throats of our loved ones, silence about the irrelevance and abuse of HIV testing. Mandatory HIV testing is already here for at least some kinds of medical treatment (pregnant women, couples undergoing fertility treatment). Some have proposed mandatory pre-marital HIV testing. What's next: Mandatory testing to receive a driver's license or passport? Chipping people with their HIV status? A positive HIV diagnosis is not only socially stigmatizing but can also be used as a devastating legal wrecking-ball, too. Thanks to critical thinkers like Duesberg, the tide is turning. When the lawsuits are done, the CDC, NIH, and the FDA will have to be dismantled. If there is a just world, then these people, the pharmaceutical industry, and the greedy, craven scientists who propagated all these lies all this time will be tried for crimes against humanity. Duesberg is a hero and should be treated as such.[26]

Anti-sex Conspiracies

Is it possible that AIDS is no more than a scare tactic to get people to stop having premarital and homosexual sex? Anti-sex conspiracies state that HIV was unleashed on gay communities as part of the rising of the religious right during the Reagan revolution, referring to AIDS as the "American Invention to Discourage Sex." Anti-sex conspiracy thinkers state that the heterosexual AIDS epidemic has been conjured to raise sexual anxiety and suppress sexuality. The anti-sex conspiracies repeatedly misuse research on HIV transmission risks to say that HIV is transmitted less than once per 1000 sex acts. The conspiracy also refutes the African sexually transmitted HIV epidemic, attributing AIDS in Africa to unclean medical practices. The pseudoscience that underlies anti-sex conspiracies was discussed in Chapter 3. The kernel of truth that underlies the anti-sex conspiracy stems from religious right and politically conservative agendas that do seem aimed at suppressing sexuality and promoting abstinence.

The political realities of AIDS are taken to an extreme level of a conspiracy that led to false claims of heterosexually transmitted HIV and "condom cops" whose sole mission is to take the pleasure out of sex. Some have even said that propagating HIV as the cause of AIDS keeps people from having "natural sex" and forcing Africans and African-Americans to use condoms to reduce the size of their population. The same type of conspiracy thinking has occurred in gay communities, as was the case in San Francisco ACTUP, which claimed AIDS was being used by the government as an instrument against the gay community. It may be that viewing AIDS as an instrument against sexuality has led sexual revolutionaries, such as those associated with *Penthouse and Hustler* magazines, to embrace denialism.

Even with as far fetched a notion that the scientific enterprise has conspired to dissuade people from having sex and to suppress Duesberg and his accomplices and the outlandish idea that HIV is only connected to AIDS so that pharmaceutical companies can sell condoms, needles, test kits and drugs, we must ultimately ask ourselves the lingering question, "what if they are right"?

What if the Denialists Are Right?

AIDS science leaves no room for musing that denialists could possibly be right in proclaiming that HIV does not cause AIDS. Tens of thousands of studies show that HIV does cause AIDS. If HIV does not cause AIDS it would mean that thousands of scientists, researchers, medical doctors, and public health officials – essentially the entire biomedical science and public health enterprise – had conspired to maintain a lie for 25 years. The notion that HIV does not exist or that the virus is harmless defies reality.

If the denialists are right, then people in Africa are dying from HIV medications and poverty, not from HIV infection. That would mean that there is something special about poverty in Africa because places with even more extreme poverty are not witnessing the death rates that are seen in Africa since AIDS. And it would mean that something odd must account for the fact that less people are dying in Brazil and Botswana since treatments for HIV became available, just as occurred in the United States and Europe. If the denialists are right, then there have been no gay men who have died of AIDS that did not either use illicit drugs or take HIV treatments. If the denialists are right it means that my friend Michael's family has been fooled because he never used heavy drugs and only tested HIV positive after he developed AIDS – long before he ever took AZT. If the denialists are right that HIV cannot be transmitted during vaginal sex (heterosexual transmission), then the more than 7,000 women and 4,000 men in 2006 in the United States who said the only risk factor they had for contracting HIV was heterosexual sex are lying. For the denialists to be right about AIDS would mean everyone else in the world is wrong, essentially meaning that the world is indeed upside-down and perhaps even flat.

Denialists are however partially correct in some of their assertions, which is a central part of the denialist ploy. Their attention to poverty as the most relevant social context of AIDS is certainly correct. But they take this fact and twist it. Poverty does not cause AIDS. Poverty encompasses numerous factors that facilitate HIV transmission including alcohol and drug abuse, poor health care, prostitution, untreated sexually transmitted infections, limited HIV testing resources, and limited HIV treatment and prevention services. There is evidence that living in a poor US neighborhood predicts HIV risks as does having insufficient food in Africa. Denialists are also correct in pointing out that there are biological co-factors for HIV and AIDS, mostly other viral infections that increase the rate of HIV disease progression to full-blown AIDS.

From the perspective of a denialist, the ramifications of being right are expressed best in terms of the AIDS establishment being wrong. One denialist told me that being right would mean being diagnosed HIV positive will no longer be giving people an emotional death sentence; no longer preventing mothers from having a natural birth; preventing people from having natural sex; separating people from society; forcing celibacy; and keeping people in committed relationships from the possibility of having a family and so on. If HIV did not case AIDS, all of these things would just go away. It is indeed unfortunate that HIV does cause AIDS.

Why Denialists Drive Scientists Crazy

Scientists are by their nature and training systematic and objective. When it comes to denialism, however, even the most renowned AIDS scientists can lose their composure. In interviews about his own reactions to Duesberg, Robert Gallo has lost his cool more than once. Gallo has talked of his amazement at the "mass ignorance coupled with the grandiosity of selling themselves as experts" displayed by the Perth Group, saying that "it would be like us arguing with Niels Bohr on quantum mechanics."[27] The same angry reactions are described by author Matt Taibbi, in his book *The Great*

Derangement. Taibbi describes investigating 9/11 conspiracy theorists, who among other things claim that the World Trade Center fell because it was pre-wired with explosives, namely "controlled demolition." When Taibbi asked structural engineers whether this was possible, they were invariably outraged by the question. Like AIDS scientists, the frustration seemed to stem from repeatedly asking a question that had been repeatedly settled expert after expert. One engineer seemed to say it best, asking "where would you go if you needed surgery? A restaurant? A bicycle shop?"[28] The point is, when we ask experts a question at the very least they expect us to believe their answer over novices.

What is it about denialists that can push a scientist out of objectivity into a fit of rage. In the Preface to this book I described my own emotional outrage to psychologist Kelly Brennan-Jones' review of Duesberg's book. In a personal sense, denialists are insulting our integrity and the value of our life's work. Referring to AIDS scientists as conspirators, frauds, Nazis and child killers is certainly personal. Even more personal are the countless colleagues, friends, and acquaintances that we have seen suffer and die of AIDS. Also maddening is that the criticisms are coming from people with little or no scientific training and universally no professional experience in AIDS.

It is easy to see why Internet blogs, open letters, and other exchanges rapidly deteriorate into name-calling and character assassinations. From the view of denialists, the exchanges confirm an irrational and non-scientific basis of the AIDS "orthodoxy." When reporters have asked one of the most vocal critics of the denialists about why he is publicly confronting their views, Cornell University AIDS scientist John Moore said:

> The reason we take these people on is because they kill people. If you persuade someone that HIV is harmless and then that person engages in unsafe sex or doesn't take effective therapies, you're killing that person. We didn't want to see any resurgence of this nonsense in the mainstream American media.[29]

The best organized response to denialism has come from a group of AIDS scientists and activists who have started their own web site www.aidstruth.org to counter denialism. Members of aidstruth.org have gone to extremes to counter denialism, including suggesting criminal action. Canadian AIDS scientist Mark Wainberg has been a target of denialism for years and ultimately concluded "As far as I'm concerned, and I hope this view is adequately represented, those who attempt to dispel the notion that HIV is the cause of AIDS are perpetrators of death. And I would very much for one like to see the Constitution of the United States and similar countries have some means in place that we can charge people who are responsible for endangering public health with charges of endangerment and bring them up on trial. I think that people like Peter Duesberg belong in jail."[30]

Anti-denialists believe that extreme actions are justified because they say there are well-accepted limits to free speech when it applies to protecting public health. Nevertheless, the general consensus is that denialists will not simply disappear. It would seem that their motivations, whether for attention, personal profit, or personal denial, will not foster a new awakening. Anti-denialists say they are acting in the public interest by attempting to remove AIDS pseudoscientists from positions of academic authority and credibility. Critics, on the other hand, say that attempting to remove people from academia for what they say is too extreme and encroaches on academic freedom. Regardless of whether you agree with these actions, they clearly illustrate the frustration that denialism is causing at least some AIDS scientists.

If denialism were merely a small number of crackpots engaged in conspiracy theories and anti-establishment blogging, they would not have the attention of some of the world's most prominent AIDS scientists. Denialists have gained attention because they have undermined public trust in medicine and have influenced the highest levels of AIDS policy makers, especially in some countries that have been hardest hit by HIV/AIDS. The impact of denialism on politics and policy is without question its most harmful device. The politics of HIV/AIDS denialism is where the most lives have truly been lost. The politics of denialism are where we now turn attention.

Politics of Denialism   **5**

The poet W.H. Auden said that true men of action in our times are not the politicians and statesmen but the scientists. I believe that's especially true when it comes to the AIDS epidemic.
President Ronald Regan, speaking for the first time about AIDS,
May 31, 1987

We have been as it were brought up on an orthodox view. Certain things that one thought one knows – HIV equals AIDS equals death. One of the things that became clear, and which was actually rather disturbing, was the fact that there was a view which was being expressed by people whose scientific credentials you can't question. I am not saying that they are necessarily correct, but it seems to me that there had been a determined effort to exclude their voice – to silence it.
President Thabo Mbeki, South Africa, Interview 2000

The AIDS crisis in America emerged out of the post-Vietnam, post-civil rights, and post-sexual revolution era. Having been organized around the civil rights struggle, gay communities were loaded with well-informed and skilled activists ready to answer the call of AIDS. One example is Chris Fons, the first AIDS activist I personally knew. Chris was born in 1968 and talked about how his mother demonstrated on nearly every social issue of the 1970s. As a young boy, Chris attended women's rights demonstrations, political rallies, and anti-war meetings, sometimes all in one day! It would seem that Chris had activism in his DNA and when he tested HIV positive he immediately became involved in the radical AIDS activist group AIDS Coalition to Unleash Power (ACTUP), soon becoming one of the most visible AIDS activists in the mid-west. Chris spoke to countless high schools about AIDS. High schools were his specialty because he may have been in his twenties, but he looked like he was in his teens. Chris died of AIDS in 1995 at the age of 27. He never did heavy drugs and he tested HIV positive well into the course of the disease, before ever taking AZT. Chris was one of thousands of young men who joined the fight against AIDS throughout the 1980s and 1990s, forcing public attention to the growing epidemic and placing AIDS on America's front pages.

Social and political activism in response to AIDS has followed a similar course in Africa. The 1960s and 1970s were also a time of social upheaval in Africa, with countries throughout the continent gaining independence from colonial rule. Coincidental with newly won freedoms and mobility, AIDS posed new threats to the populace. Freedom came later to the Republic of South Africa, as did AIDS. Like the first AIDS activists in the United States, South African AIDS activists were born from those who actively fought against the Apartheid regime. Most notably, the Treatment Action Campaign (TAC), modeled after ACTUP, battled the very government it fought to elect in an effort to gain access to HIV testing and antiretroviral therapies, a battle that continued well into the coming decade.

HIV/AIDS is as complex socially, or perhaps even more complex, as it is biologically. The nature of HIV infection demands open and frank discussions about sex and sexuality, confronting addictions and facing the death of young people. Sex, drugs, and youth have also helped to make AIDS a political football. And so it goes, the politics of AIDS is inextricably tied to denialism. Presidents who have said nothing about AIDS, presidents who have said that HIV is not the cause of AIDS, and presidents who have claimed they can cure AIDS have all fueled denialism in their countries and beyond. Here we examine the politics of HIV/AIDS in its close relationship to denialism.

The Press Conference

The single most significant political event in the history of AIDS may well have taken place on April 23, 1984. On that date, Robert Gallo and then US Department of Health and Human Services (HHS) Secretary Margaret Heckler under President Reagan told the world of the discovery of the virus that causes AIDS. Breaking from the usual order of events, the press conference took place in advance of the scientific publications documenting the discovery. The urgency to identify the agent causing AIDS likely overrode any such formality. After all, the articles had undergone peer review and were in the process of being published. Still, media announcements are supposed to follow the publication of scientific findings, not precede them. Surely other mistakes were made, including suggesting that a vaccine against HIV was only two years away. In a 2006 interview, Margaret Heckler recounted the press conference in this way:

We announced the identification of the virus, and that was a tremendously important announcement on the part of HHS and Dr. Gallo. At that time, this is the place where I do feel, obviously, that I misjudged. I worked with Dr. Gallo because he was briefing me constantly, as everyone was, and I have so much confidence in him, and so much respect for him. He had identified the human T-Cell leukemia virus. He had a track record that was impressive. We anticipated the subject about a vaccine. When would a vaccine be available? was the question. I listened to, again, the leaders of the department, who said they really didn't know, and I asked Bob Gallo, "What do you think?" and he said two years. In the press conference, I did say two years, and that turned out to be totally incorrect. But at that time, we did not know that the replication of the virus would be so difficult – and it still is a problem. It was a scientific fact that had not ever entered the picture before.[1]

The controversy that followed the press conference embroiled Gallo and may very well have cost him a Nobel Prize. Indeed, the controversy over whether Gallo or his French counterparts actually discovered the virus plagues him to this day. Ultimately, the French and US governments worked out a settlement for the co-discovery of HIV and the patent rights for the HIV antibody test. Still, it is The Press Conference that has come to symbolize AIDS science in the eyes of denialists. Duesberg emphasizes the historical significance of the Press Conference when he talks about AIDS, as seen in the following except:

The period of research into the cause of AIDS in which both infectious and non-infectious agents were considered lasted only three years. It started with the identification of AIDS in 1981 and officially ended in April 1984 with the announcement of the 'AIDS virus' at an international press conference conducted by the secretary of Health and Human Services and the federal AIDS researcher Robert Gallo in Washington, DC. This announcement was made prior to the publication of any scientific evidence confirming the virus theory. With this unprecedented maneuver, Gallo's discovery bypassed review by the scientific community. Science by press conference was substituted for the conventional process of scientific validation, which is based on publications in the professional literature. The "AIDS virus" became instant national dogma, and the tremendous weight of federal resources was diverted into just one race – the race to study the AIDS virus.[2]

Nearly every denialist book, brochure and Internet web site highlights The Press Conference as a reason to question whether HIV causes AIDS. Some denialists are so obsessed with The Press Conference the Rethinking AIDS Society declared April 23rd International Rethinking AIDS Day, a holiday for the world to remember The Press Conference. Denialists proclaim that once announced as the virus that causes AIDS, there was no looking back, saying that by virtue of The Press Conference, the science of HIV equals AIDS was forever sealed. All alternative theories of AIDS were discarded, putting into place a global bandwagon that every scientist, except Duesberg and a few other dissidents, jumped on. The following excepts provide a sense for just how important The Press Conference remains in the fiber of denialism.

- Denialist Organization Alive and Well: "On April 23, 1984, Gallo called an international press conference in conjunction with the US Department of Health and Human Services (HHS). He used this forum to announce his discovery of a new retrovirus described as 'the probable cause of AIDS.' Although Gallo presented no evidence to support his tentative assumption, the HHS immediately characterized it as 'another miracle of American medicine...the triumph of science over a dreaded disease.' "[3]
- Seth Roberts, Psychology Professor at UC Berkeley: "Just before the publication of the *Science* papers, then-secretary of Health and Human Services, Margaret Heckler held a press conference starring Gallo. She proclaimed, 'Today we add a new miracle to the long honor roll of American medicine and science' – a bit of puffery not quite consistent with Gallo's current claim that he and Heckler gave the French 'full credit.' "[4]
- Denialist journalist Liam Scheff: "It was a new retrovirus called HTLV-III (later re-named HIV). Later that same day, he patented the modified cell-line he'd originally gotten from Montagnier. He hadn't published a single word of his research. Robert Gallo, a government-backed scientist, simply announced that a retroviral-epidemic was on its way."[5]

The Press Conference, by its very nature, provided the first bridge between AIDS science and AIDS politics. Nevertheless, President Reagan publicly ignored AIDS for the first six years of the US epidemic. Although AIDS emerged on his watch, President Reagan turned away from AIDS. In the context of a conservative presidency backed by the Religious Right, the announcement at the press conference was fertile ground for mistrust and conspiracy theorizing. Questions of scientific misconduct around the discovery of the virus and suggesting a vaccine was forthcoming certainly did not help matters. Scientists and politicians have held many press conferences since 1984 and many have made regrettable promises. For example, more than ten years after the Gallo/Heckler press conference, President Clinton called for a concerted effort to develop an AIDS vaccine within a decade. Contrary to President Kennedy's challenge to put a man on the moon within a decade, there was no scientific basis to say that an HIV vaccine could be accomplished in that timeframe. In fact, it proved easier to go to the moon than find an HIV vaccine. Just as public confidence in the space program grew from the successes in the Apollo space program, public confidence in AIDS science has eroded and denialism is emboldened with every failed vaccine. Duesberg himself said to me in a single breath that failing to find a vaccine proves that "AIDS is not caused by an infectious agent." Most every denialist exploits the failed predictions of AIDS science, summed up by their saying,

"More than twenty years after a cure for AIDS was promised to have arrived, there is none, and there likely never will be a vaccine."[6] Statements with elements of the truth that are easily conjured into denialist rhetoric.

Presidential Denialism

In 1981, the first AIDS cases were diagnosed in New York and California. It was the first year of the new Reagan presidency. Ronald Reagan's silence about AIDS is shamefully legendary. Backed by rightwing religious and conservative groups that denounce homosexuality, such as Jerry Falwell's Moral Majority, President Reagan did not mention the word AIDS in public until asked about increasing research funding for AIDS during a press conference in September 1985:

> Q. Mr. President, the Nation's best-known AIDS scientist says the time has come now to boost existing research into what he called a minor moon-shot program to attack this AIDS epidemic that has struck fear into the Nation's health workers and even its schoolchildren. Would you support a massive government research program against AIDS like the one that President Nixon launched against cancer?
>
> *President Reagan.* I have been supporting it for more than 4 years now. It's been one of the top priorities with us, and over the last 4 years, and including what we have in the budget for '86, it will amount to over a half a billion dollars that we have provided for research on AIDS in addition to what I'm sure other medical groups are doing. And we have $100 million in the budget this year; it'll be 126 million next year. So, this is a top priority with us. Yes, there's no question about the seriousness of this and the need to find an answer.
>
> Q. If I could follow up, sir. The scientist who talked about this, who does work for the Government, is in the National Cancer Institute. He was referring to your program and the increase that you proposed as being not nearly enough at this stage to go forward and really attack the problem.
>
> *President Reagan.* I think with our budgetary constraints and all, it seems to me that $126 million in a single year for research has got to be something of a vital contribution.[7]

The second time President Reagan spoke of AIDS was in his message to the Congress on America's Agenda for the Future in February 1986, where he said,

> We will continue, as a high priority, the fight against Acquired Immune Deficiency Syndrome (AIDS). An unprecedented research effort is underway to deal with this

major epidemic public health threat. The number of AIDS cases is expected to increase. While there are hopes for drugs and vaccines against AIDS, none is immediately at hand. Consequently, efforts should focus on prevention, to inform and to lower risks of further transmission of the AIDS virus. To this end, I am asking the Surgeon General to prepare a report to the American people on AIDS.[8]

It was not until May 1987 that President Reagan would deliver his first full address on AIDS. Speaking at a dinner of the newly established American Foundation for AIDS Research (AmFAR) at the invitation of founder Elizabeth Taylor, the President spoke of the tragedy of AIDS and the discrimination that people who had AIDS were encountering. In the history of AIDS, President Reagan will be remembered for what he did not say over the course of 6 years during which nearly 30,000 Americans had been diagnosed with AIDS and unknown numbers of people were infected with HIV.

Among heads of State, President Reagan is certainly not alone. Openly addressing AIDS comes with a political price tag. Like Reagan, Nelson Mandela did not make AIDS a priority in the new and free South Africa, and like Reagan who delegated AIDS to Vice President George H. Bush, Mandela delegated AIDS to his Vice President Thabo Mbeki. History has also shown that the next US President, George H. Bush, paid a political price for taking action against AIDS, making him appear as "pandering to gays." Mandela now speaks frankly about AIDS and his regret for not making AIDS a priority in his presidency. Nelson Mandela is honest about his discomfort speaking publicly about sex, reflecting the general social taboos against open sexual discourse in many cultures. Tragically, Mandela's own son Makgatho Mandela died of AIDS in 2005.

Denialism at the top of governments has been observed throughout the history of AIDS. In the 1990s, Russia was experiencing its first major outbreaks of HIV/AIDS among injection drug users. Yet the Russian government failed to act in prevention and treatment. Similarly, China ignored HIV as it rapidly spread through injection drug use, prostitution, and blood plasma trade. By contrast, Presidents who directly confronted the onslaught of AIDS acted to save countless lives of their citizens. It is widely held that Thailand and Uganda both stemmed significant loss of life to AIDS because their governments excised the moral authority to enact bold HIV prevention programs.

Considerable ignorance on AIDS has also been demonstrated by men who are well within reach of the presidency. For example, in the 2004 vice presidential candidates debate, Vice President Dick Cheney was asked the question, "Black women between the ages of 25 and 44 are 13 times more likely to die of the disease (AIDS) than their counterparts' in this country. What should the government's role be in helping to end the growth of this epidemic?" The vice president of the United States, who had been in the job for four years and was seeking re-election amazingly responded, "I have not heard those numbers with respect to African-American women. I was not aware that it was – that they're in epidemic."[9]

In the 2008 presidential election, Senator John McCain, while campaigning for the Presidential nomination was asked "Should U.S. taxpayer money go to places like Africa to fund contraception to prevent AIDS?" Senator McCain replied, "Well I think it's a combination. The guy I really respect on this is [Senator] Dr. Coburn. He believes – and I was just reading the thing he wrote – that you should do what you can to encourage abstinence where there is going to be sexual activity. Where that doesn't succeed, then he thinks that we should employ contraceptives as well. But I agree with him that the first priority is on abstinence. I look to people like Dr. Coburn. I'm not very wise on it. I haven't thought about it. Before I give you an answer, let me think about it. Let me think about it a little bit because I never got a question about it before. I don't know if I would use taxpayers' money for it." The reporter followed up asking "What about grants for sex education in the United States? Should they include instructions about using contraceptives? Or should it be Bush's policy, which is just abstinence?" After a long pause, the man who was seeking the office of the Presidency responded "Ahhh. I think I support the president's policy." The reporter continued on and asked, "So no contraception, no counseling on contraception. Just abstinence. Do you think contraceptives help stop the spread of HIV?" McCain answered "You've stumped me. Are we on the Straight Talk express? I'm not informed enough on it. Let me find out. You know, I'm sure I've taken a position on it on the past. I have to find out what my position was. Brian [a McCain aide], would you find out what my position is on contraception – I'm sure I'm opposed to government spending on it, I'm sure I support the president's policies on it."[10]

In South Africa, Deputy President Jacob Zuma led the country's AIDS Task Force and in 2006 was brought up on charges for sexually assaulting an HIV positive woman. He denied the charge and won his trial, during which he stated that he had consensual sex with the woman and showered afterward to reduce his risk for being infected with HIV. In 2007, Jacob Zuma became the President of the African National Congress, placing him in position to be South Africa's next president.[11]

Presidential AIDS Advisors

Presidential Advisory Councils reveal the political views of any presidential administration's AIDS policies. The first Presidential AIDS Panel was appointed by President Reagan in 1987. The Chairman of the Reagan Presidential AIDS Panel was Dr. Eugene Mayberry from the Mayo Clinic. By 1987, there were several physicians and scientists working on AIDS, a growing cadre of experts. Still, Reagan appointed a doctor who had no experience with AIDS. Upon his appointment, Mayberry said "I'm no AIDS expert. I do, as a physician, know a little bit about it, have kept up a little with it, and I do know it's a great problem of national concern."[12] Another member of the Reagan AIDS Panel was Theresa Crenshaw, a sex therapist who supported removing children with AIDS from public schools, despite the fact that it was well established that HIV infected children posed no threat to other children and were in no way at risk themselves.

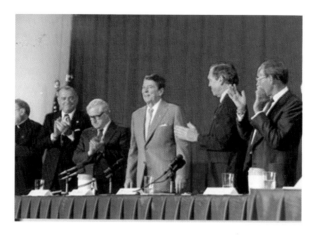

Photo 5.1 President Ronald Reagan, HHS Secretary Otis R. Bowen, Dr. James B. Wyngaarden and members of the Commission on the Human Immunodeficiency Virus Epidemic
Source: National Institutes of Health

President Clinton's Advisory Council Chair was Scott Hitt, a Beverly Hills physician who years later surrendered his license to practice medicine in California due to allegations of sexually molesting two patients at his medical office. During the Clinton years, there were huge increases in AIDS funding, expansion of treatment, prevention, and care. Yet a federal ban on providing access to sterile injection supplies to prevent the spread of HIV among drug users persisted in the face of science. The failure to legalize access to needles and syringes was purely political, running against all scientific evidence and public health interests. A panel of leading scientists assembled by the National Institutes of Health in 1996 formulated the consensus that:

> An impressive body of evidence suggests powerful effects from needle exchange programs. The number of studies showing beneficial effects on behaviors such as needle sharing greatly outnumbers those showing no effects. There is no longer doubt that these programs work, yet there is a striking disjunction between what science dictates and what policy delivers.[13]

The science had definitively answered all concerns that had been raised about needle exchange programs. Does needle exchange promote drug use? No. Time and again research showed that there was either no change or decreased drug use after needle exchange programs were implemented. Do needle exchange programs encourage non-drug users to use drugs? No. After implementing needle exchange programs there had been no evidence that community norms change in favor of drug use or that more people begin using drugs. Do needle exchange programs increase the number of discarded needles in the community? No. In the majority of studies, there is no increase in used needles discarded in public places. The panel of scientists therefore recommended lifting the federal ban on needle exchange programs to prevent the spread of HIV. It did not happen.

Nearly every science-based public health organization joined the call to lift the federal ban on clean syringe access, including the American Medical Association, the American Public Health Association, and the New York Academy of Medicine, as well as major medical schools from Yale University to the University of Hawaii. The ban still was not lifted, refuting science and demonstrating a policy of denialism.

Senator Thomas Coburn (R), a family practice physician from Oklahoma, chaired President George W. Bush's Presidential Advisory Council on HIV/AIDS. Senator Coburn had been involved in AIDS policy for some time prior to serving as Chair of the President's Advisory Council. Coburn has a strong stand on abstinence-based programs for HIV prevention, proclaiming, "Condoms do not prevent most STDs" and that "safe" sex is a myth. Also among President Bush's AIDS Advisors was Dr. Joseph McIlhaney, a Texas doctor known for rejecting the use of condoms to prevent the spread of HIV and other sexually transmitted diseases. Like Senator Coburn, Dr. McIllheney strongly supports abstinence-only programs for HIV prevention. The official HIV/AID prevention policy of the Bush administration had been the hierarchically ordered acronym ABC – Abstinence, Be Faithful, Condoms. That is, abstain from sex outside marriage, be faithful to your spouse, and otherwise use condoms. All federally funded AIDS prevention required including an ABC approach in their programs. In the President's Emergency Plan for AIDS Relief (PEPFAR), a major program that provides AIDS resources to the developing world, there was a requirement that two out of three dollars for prevention be spent on abstinence/being faithful (A/B-only) programming.

The science of AIDS prevention leaves little room for doubt that abstinence only prevention programs simply do not work in reducing sexual risk behaviors. Abstinence-only programming places policy at odds with science because it ignores overwhelming evidence that prevention programs that emphasize condom use are effective in reducing risks for HIV. Abstinence-only programs cannot be scientifically justified, and yet the prevailing public

health policies are abstinence-based. The ABC prevention message is prominent in countries that accept US funding for AIDS prevention, most notably
Uganda, where President Yoweri Museveni strongly endorsed the ABC message. As I noted earlier, Uganda had experienced among the lowest rates of
AIDS in the 1990s, far lower than any of its neighbors in Africa. However,
Uganda's prevention success occurred well before the ABC policy was in
place. Remarkably, subsequent implementation of ABC messages in Uganda
was followed by increases in HIV/AIDS. Other countries, such as Brazil, have
refused US aide because of mandates for abstinence programming and
requirements to outlaw prostitution.

Do presidential advisory panels really advise Presidents? Or, do presidential panels serve as political cover for partisan policies? The Union of Concerned Scientists released a report in 2004 entitled *Scientific Integrity in
Policymaking* claiming that "President Bush intentionally appointed under-
qualified individuals to his AIDS Advisory Council as part of an effort to
manipulate the government's scientific advisory system." As often is the case,
the Council was intended to present the appearance of expert advice while
controlling the advice given. The 2002 Presidential Advisory Council held
only two meetings and issued five recommendations to President Bush
contrasted with the 597 recommendations offered by the 1988 AIDS commission to President Reagan. Throughout the history of AIDS, presidents have
selected advisors who are consistent with the positions of their political
constituencies rather than informed by science. No presidential AIDS advisory panel, however, has been as blatantly AIDS denialistic as that of President Thabo Mbeki of South Africa.

Debunking Myths About AIDS in Africa

The AIDS epidemic in Africa originated in the central region and spread
southward through migration and commerce routes. The major mode of HIV
transmission in Africa remains vaginal intercourse. Why has HIV spread
through the general heterosexual population in Africa unlike anywhere else
in the world? The spread of HIV/AIDS in African is not a mystery. The factors
that account for AIDS in Africa are no different than those that account for
AIDS everywhere, namely people in close networks becoming exposed to
HIV infected blood and sexual fluids. One of the most important factors in
the spread of HIV is the types of sexual partnerships that people have. For
example, HIV spreads fastest when people have more than one sex partner in
a short time period, called concurrent sex partnerships. HIV spreads most
rapidly when a newly infected person has multiple sex partners who then

become infected and they themselves have multiple concurrent partners. Also critical in Africa's AIDS epidemics are co-epidemics of other sexually transmitted infections, particularly herpes simplex virus infection because it creates recurrent open sores on the genitals. Another factor in the spread of HIV is older men having sex with younger partners. Older men are more likely to have HIV, resist condom use, and have sex with multiple younger partners. These same risk factors, concurrent sex partners, co-epidemics of other sexually transmitted infections, and inter-generational sex account for the rapid spread of HIV in Africa, the Caribbean, as well as gay communities in the United States, Europe, and Latin America.

AIDS as a disease is also no different in Africa than anywhere else in the world. HIV destroys the immune system the same in Africans just as it does in non-Africans. Africans with AIDS may suffer different opportunistic illnesses when their immune system fails simply because they live in places with different disease causing agents. For example, people in the United States are more likely exposed to the virus that causes Kaposi's Sarcoma (KS) whereas people in Africa are more likely exposed to Tuberculosis. It is also a myth that HIV and AIDS are diagnosed differently in Africa than in other parts of the world. Today people throughout the world are tested for HIV when they are suspected of having AIDS.

Apartheid, AIDS, and Freedom

Just as HIV was making its way down the African continent to the Republic of South Africa, the country was being transformed from the white minority ruled Apartheid government to a true democracy. In 1990, newly elected President Nelson Mandela reformed all facets of his country while healing the wounds left by decades of racial injustice. President Mandela and his African National Congress (ANC) focused on poverty as the most critical social problem requiring immediate attention. Placing poverty at the center of the ANC's agenda was consistent with their official AIDS policy, strongly emphasizing the social and cultural aspects of the HIV/AIDS epidemic, while downplaying the viral and behavioral aspects. Focusing on poverty and revamping a neglected health care system was the clear AIDS policy in South Africa throughout the 1990s.

President Mandela delegated the national AIDS policy to then Deputy President Thabo Mbeki who later became South Africa's second freely elected president. By many accounts, President Mbeki is a highly intelligent man. Since 1990 South Africa's economy has soared to new heights. Today South Africa has a gross domestic product (GDP) that is four times that of its neighbors, comprising nearly 25% of the GDP of the entire African continent. South Africa accounts for nearly half of all of Africa's industrial output and produces half of the continent's electricity. The number of South Africans living in poverty has dropped continuously each year since the early 1990s, down from 52% in 1999 to 47% in 2004 and to 43% by 2007. Since 1995, South Africa has built more than 2 million homes, provided new electricity to more than 3 million homes, and provided clean water for the first-time to over 16 million homes.

At once while South Africa's economy and standard of living improved, poverty declined and yet the country experienced the growth of a devastating HIV/AIDS epidemic. The AIDS statistics in South Africa are cold and stark. Today, an estimated 800 people die of AIDS each day in South Africa and another 1000 are infected with HIV. In 2006, 29% of pregnant women attending antenatal clinics were HIV infected. The dramatic increase in HIV prevalence among South African women went from virtually no HIV present among women in 1990 to one in three women testing HIV positive in 2004. A 2005 nationally representative survey estimated that 11% of all South Africans over 2 years old were living with HIV/AIDS, with the rate increasing to 16% for persons between the ages of 15 and 49 years old. The head of South Africa's Medical Research Council estimates that AIDS had killed 336,000 South Africans between 2005 and 2006. The annual number of registered deaths in South Africa rose by 87%, again this was during a time when poverty

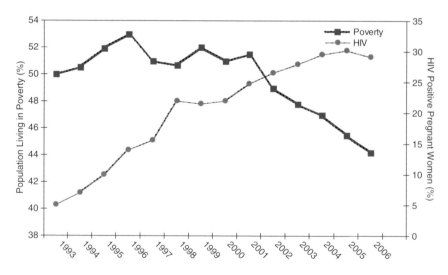

Fig. 5.1 Poverty rates and HIV infections among pregnant women in South Africa, 1993–2006
Sources: Poverty data van der Berg et al., University of Stellenbosch, 2007; HIV infection data Journal-AIDS, University of the Witwatersrand, 2007

rates were declining. Among those aged 25–49 years, the rise in deaths was 169%. Although more people may have died simply because population growth was also occurring, population growth is not a plausible explanation for the greatest increase in deaths occurring among young people. In 1997, 25–49 year olds accounted for 30% of all deaths, whereas in 2005 42% of all deaths occurred in this age group. These population based statistics clearly support the corresponding HIV prevalence statistics and reflect HIV as the obvious cause of AIDS. The increasing AIDS deaths that occurred while poverty decreased, even as antiretrovirals were rolled out in 2003, also runs completely counter to the Duesbergian notion that poverty and HIV treatments cause AIDS. Figure 5.1 shows the declining rates of poverty in South Africa between 1993 and 2006, juxtaposed to the escalating HIV/AIDS cases during those same years.

South Africa and State Denialism

Perhaps South Africa was particularly vulnerable to denialism. South African suspicion about a disease that was killing more blacks than whites may have been inevitable following the ruthless wrath of colonialism and Apartheid. President Mbeki expressed his belief that a conspiracy exists to advance HIV as the cause of AIDS. In his biography of the President, Mark Gevisser states that Mbeki believes that South Africans who espouse the orthodox view that HIV causes AIDS, including Nelson Mandela, the labor unions, as well as AIDS scientists are financially beholden to drug companies. Gevisser also writes of how President Mbeki has expressed concern that his life could be threatened by western governments and the pharmaceutical industry because of his opposition to antiretroviral medications.

Denialism has plagued South Africa nearly as badly as the epidemic itself. Early in his Presidency, Mbeki became involved in a failed attempt to develop a treatment for AIDS called Virodene. In a complex series of events, President Mbeki backed the African development of the drug, which has an industrial solvent as its primary ingredient. As it turned out, Virodene demonstrated no benefit and has become mired in scandal regarding its finances.

In the year 2000, South Africa hosted the International AIDS Conference in the seaside city of Durban. In his opening address to world leaders in AIDS research, Mbeki emphasized poverty as the greatest threat to his country and spoke minimally about AIDS:

> The world's biggest killer and the greatest cause of ill-health and suffering across the globe are listed almost at the end of the International Classification of Diseases. It is given the code Z59.5 – extreme poverty. Poverty is the main reason why babies

are not vaccinated, why clean water and sanitation are not provided, why curative drugs and other treatments are unavailable and why mothers die in childbirth. It is the underlying cause of reduced life expectancy, handicap, disability and starvation. Poverty is a major contributor to mental illness, stress, suicide, family disintegration and substance abuse. Every year in the developing world 12.2 million children under 5 years die, most of them from causes which could be prevented for just a few US cents per child. They die largely because of world indifference, but most of all they die because they are poor.[14]

Thus, the speech that was seen as an opportunity to place South Africa on the world map of AIDS priorities was lost because Mbeki turned away from AIDS toward poverty. In 2000 Mbeki also convened his Presidential AIDS Advisory Panel, which had over 30 members. Remarkably, nearly half of the "experts" were denialists including Peter Duesberg, Harvey Bialy, Etienne De Harven, Roberto Giraldo, Klaus Koehnlein, Eleni Papadopulos-Eleopulos, David Rasnick, Gordon Stewart, and Val Turner. Mbeki did not come directly out publicly saying that HIV does not cause AIDS, but he also has not said that he believes HIV does cause AIDS. In his biography of the President, Gevisser tells how Mbeki regrets having withdrawn himself from the "AIDS debate." He states that members of his government who were concerned that South Africa was suffering international repercussions from Mbeki's views on AIDS, including from his silence at the Durban AIDS conference, and pressured him to step back from the issue.

Mbeki refutes the idea that HIV/AIDS is the major killer in Africa and believes that AIDS detracts from the real problems Africans face in unemployment, racism, and globalization. He has said that he has personally not known anyone who has died of AIDS, despite members of his own government openly dying of the disease. Some speculate that Mbeki must mean that he has known people who may have died of antiretroviral medications, but not of AIDS. His conviction is that the established science cannot be trusted and must be considered mixed and inconclusive. In his opening remarks to his AIDS Advisory panel in May of 2000, Mbeki expressed his views on AIDS, leaving little doubt about his denialist beliefs:

We were looking for answers because all of the information that has been communicated points to the reality that we are faced with a catastrophe, and you can't respond to a catastrophe merely by saying I will do what is routine. You have to respond to a catastrophe in a way that recognizes that you are facing a catastrophe. And here we are talking about people – it is not death of animal stock or something like that, but people. Millions and millions of people. Somewhat of a storm broke out around this question, which in truth took me by surprise. There is an approach that asks why this President of South Africa is trying to give legitimacy to discredited scientists, because after all, all the questions of science concerning this matter had been resolved by the year 1984. I don't know of any science that gets resolved in that manner with a cut-off year beyond which science does not develop any further. It sounds like a biblical absolute truth and I do not imagine that science consists of biblical absolute truths. There was this very strong response saying: don't do this. I have seen even in the last few days, a scientist who I'm quite certain is eminent who said that perhaps the best thing to do is that we should lock up some of these dissidents in jail and that would shut them up. It is a very peculiar response but it seemed to me to suggest that it must surely be because people are exceedingly worried by the fact that large numbers of people are dying. In that context any suggestion whatsoever that dealing with this is being postponed because somebody is busy looking at some obscure scientific theory, is seen as a betrayal of people. Perhaps that is why you had that kind of response which sought to say: let us freeze scientific discourse at a particular point; and let those who do not agree with the mainstream be isolated and not spoken to. Indeed, it seems implied that one of the important measures to judge whether a scientific view is correct is to count numbers: how many scientists are on this side of the issue and how many are on the other – if the majority are on this side, and then this must be correct.[15]

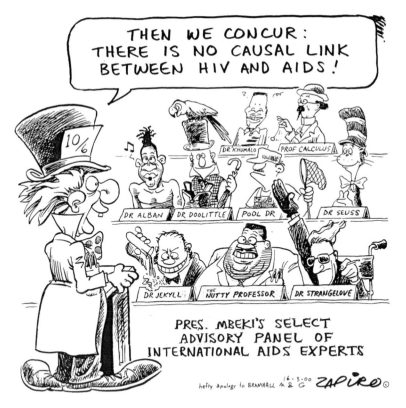

Display 5.1 South Africa's political cartoonist Zapiro's depiction of the 2000 South African Presidential AIDS Panel. I searched widely for an actual photograph of the panel and I am convinced none exists

President Mbeki became the center of international outrage for his embracing denialism. Making what he describes as one of the most difficult [decisions] of his long political career, Mbeki withdrew from the public AIDS "debate." Andrew Feinstein, a former member of the African National Congress and Member of Parliament, recalls the day that Mbeki announced to his party that he would be withdrawing from discussions on AIDS. The President was visibly upset and affirmed his personal questioning of whether HIV causes AIDS.[16] After Mbeki removed himself from the "AIDS debate," he relied on top policy officials to manage the problem. Next to President Mbeki, the most destructive person in terms of South African AIDS policy was Health Minister Dr. Manto Tshabalala-Msimang. University of Cape Town Economics Professor Nicoli Nattrass provides a detailed account of the Health Minister's role in blocking antiretroviral medications, especially to prevent HIV transmission from mothers to infants. The Health Minister's AIDS policies emphasize the potential side effects of treatments while ignoring their benefits. In her book *Mortal Combat: AIDS Denialism and the Struggle for Antiretrovirals in South Africa*, Nattrass also presents a history of the Treatment Action Campaign (TAC), South Africa's activist movement that has countered the denialist policies of Mbeki and Minster Tshabalala-Msimang.

South Africa's Health Minister, commonly called with all due respect by her first name Manto, repeatedly rejects the use of antiretroviral medications for treating people with HIV/AIDS and for preventing HIV transmission from HIV infected women to their babies. She has been closely advised by pseudoscientist and vitamin pushers Roberto Giraldo and Matthias Rath, advocating nutritional approaches to treating HIV/AIDS. She has also embraced the pseudoscience that claims successful treatment of AIDS by vitamins in what Nathan Gefften from TAC has called state sponsored pseudoscience. As discussed earlier, David Rasnick and Matthias Rath performed those unethical and unlawful studies of mega-dose vitamins for treating HIV/AIDS in South Africa providing bogus evidence to the Health Ministry. Rath has publicly acclaimed "The Dr. Rath Health Foundation Africa has the support of our Minister of Health and our Government. The vitamin programs used are qualified as food and nutrition. As opposed to toxic ARV drugs, these programs are safe because they are natural. Don't fall for the dirty tricks of the Drug Cartel: trust our Government and those who support it."[17] The South African government did not deny or take action against these statements. In fact, there is considerable evidence that the government promoted AIDS pseudoscience while it also provided credibility to denialists. Manto openly proclaims that HIV treatments are toxic poison, stating in 2003 "In my heart I believe it is not right to hand them [AZT and other ARV drugs] out to my people."[18]

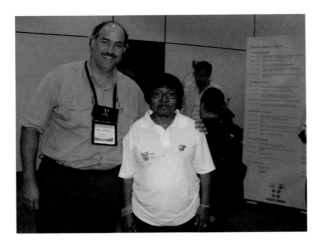

Photo 5.2 I met the South African Minister of Health Manto Tshabalala-Msimang at the International AIDS Conference in Toronto 2006

Eric Goemaere head of Médecins Sans Frontières spoke of Rath and his relationship to Manto in an interview for the medical journal *The Lancet:* In this interview, Goemaere said "This guy [Rath] is killing people by luring them with unrecognized treatment without any scientific evidence." Goemaere quoted the statistic that one-third of new AIDS patients who come to South African clinics present at very late stages of disease despite door-to-door campaigns encouraging people to seek treatment early. He said, "There is no doubt about it that people are trying alternatives to ARVs because they are afraid of the side-effects and Rath is one of the big alternatives."[19] South Africa's Treatment Action Campaign has repeatedly documented government support for Rath and has filed numerous legal actions against the Health Ministry.[20]

In 2006, Manto fell seriously ill, ultimately requiring a liver transplant. During her absence, her Deputy Health Minister Nozizwe Madlala-Routledge assumed leadership of the Health Ministry. By all accounts, Deputy Minister Madlala-Routledge was progressive and accepted the benefits of treating HIV/AIDS with antiretroviral drugs. She was certainly a maverick compared to her ailing superior, having publicly taken an HIV test and made several public statements supportive of HIV treatments. Ultimately, the Deputy Minister was prohibited from speaking publicly about AIDS. Still, she continued to be outspoken. In a most noteworthy action, Madlala-Routledge angered her superiors in the Mbeki's administration when she declared the rates of infant mortality in South African hospitals due to HIV/AIDS a national emergency.

Deputy Minister Madlala-Routledge also held the leadership role in constructing the country's new national strategic AIDS plan, bringing great hope and optimism to the country. After the Health Minister recovered and returned from medical leave to her post, Deputy Minister Madlala-Routledge was astonishingly fired by President Mbeki. This action was seen as yet more evidence for Mbeki's denialism and were again met with international outrage.

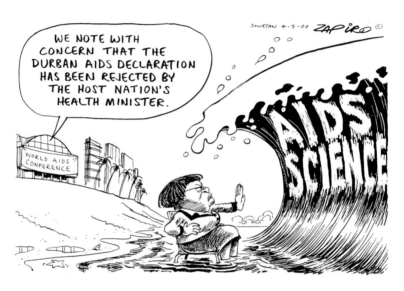

Display 5.2 South Africa's political cartoonist Zapiro's depiction of the Health Minister rebuking AIDS science at the 2000 International AIDS Conference held in Durban South Africa

In a rare response, President Mbeki released an explanation for his actions. In his statement, he continued to raise his belief that HIV treatments require "rigorous scientific testing," leaving little doubt that Mbeki remains a denialist. In fact, the denialists have designated him their most honorable member of the movement. The homepage to "virusmyth" posts a petition for AIDS Rethinkers to sign in support of President Mbeki. In 2003, The Alberta Reappraising AIDS Society awarded the Superior AIDS Rethinking Action Honor to President Mbeki. The citation for the award reads,

> Thabo Mbeki, the President of South Africa, has never claimed that HIV does not cause AIDS. But, simply by asking for an investigation into the question, he has managed to turn the entire AIDS establishment against him. The catechism of AIDS, the 'Durban Declaration', was aimed squarely at him by people who think that it is just as wrong for politicians to ask questions as for scientists.[21]

The all consuming question is why? Why would President Mbeki, an otherwise seemingly intelligent man come to embrace denialism? From a distance, one might assume it was the cost of the drugs. With an overwhelming number of people with HIV/AIDS to care for, perhaps it was the financial burdens of treatment on balance with other priorities that led him astray? But there is no evidence that Mbeki was merely hiding behind a cloak of denialism to avoid the cost of HIV treatments. In fact, there is ample evidence that providing HIV treatments would have saved South Africa's money by preventing costly illnesses and reducing the number of infected babies. Economist Nicoli Nattrass has done extensive analyses that show the cost of providing treatment in South Africa is offset by reducing worker absenteeism, raising productivity, raising household incomes, and potentially reducing rates of HIV transmission.[22] In addition, South Africa had turned away efforts to bring in HIV treatments at low cost as well as donated drugs. Money was apparently not the motive for Mbeki's denialism.

Two recent biographical works help shed light on Mbeki's turning to denialism, Mark Gevisser's 2007 biography of the president and Andrew Feinstein's memoirs of his years in government. Gevisser writes that the political context of AIDS in South Africa helps explain the inroads for denialism into politics. As South Africa emerged out of the apartheid era in 1990, the great hope for a new society was not about to be derailed by a new disease. A decade later both domestic and international forces pressured Mbeki to deal with the growing AIDS problem. In particular, the 2000 International AIDS Conference would focus the world's attention on South Africa and the country's response to the epidemic.

Prior to the Durban AIDS Conference, in 1999 President Mbeki received an extensive file of AIDS denialist materials. Assembled by Johannesburg journalist Anita Allen and attorney Anthony Brink, the dossier filled with AIDS denialist writings is said to have brought Mbeki to question the medical and scientific basis for HIV as the cause of AIDS. Brink is quoted as saying that he directly introduced Mbeki to denialism, stating that it is worth telling his story of "how a lone radical activist lawyer had blocked the world's largest pharmaceutical corporation and turned South Africa's president and health minister adamantly and vocally against its popular drug." Mbeki's initial exposure to denialism is also said to have come through seeking out information from Duesberg associate David Rasnick.[23] After speaking with Rasnick Mbeki is said to have then turned to the Internet where he became absorbed in learning as much about AIDS as he could, unfiltered and regardless of the source. His reliance on his own intellect along with his suspicion of the west, medicine, Big Pharma, and others for information left Mbeki vulnerable to Duesbergian accounts of AIDS. Mbeki particularly revolted against the notion that AIDS originated in Africa and that sexual behaviors of Africans would spread the disease any differently than anywhere else. His misperception seems to have been that the blame Africans were receiving for AIDS stemmed from old myths about African sexuality. The denialists also appealed to Mbeki because they attacked the notion that AIDS was sexually transmitted. From his own interpretation of AIDS science, his discussions with denialists, and the denialist literature that he accessed on the Internet, Mbeki astonishingly came to believe that there was a censoring of alternative views on AIDS and there deserved to be an actual debate about whether HIV causes AIDS.

Much of South Africa's AIDS policies under Mbeki appear rooted in a 133 page document that was circulated in the South African government in early 2002. The document was produced anonymously, although many believe that Mbeki himself had a hand in writing it. The style of writing is chaotic, rambling, and unconnected, resembling some of the writings produced by South African attorney Anthony Brink. Referred to as the *Castro-Hlongwane, Caravans, Cats, Geese, Foot & Mouth, and Statistics* document, there are descriptions of how AIDS promotes stereotypes of Africans as sexually primitive and insatiable. The *Castro Hlongwane* document talks about how poverty is the world's biggest killer and how rapidly changing societies face risks if the lower social strata becomes overly indulgent. The Marxist overtones of *Castro-Hlongware* were thought to reflect president Mbeki's own political philosophy which was clearly influenced by the years he spent in exile in Russia.

The *Castro-Hlongware* attacks South Africa's earliest and most prominent AIDS scientists in an effort to discredit them. For example, Salim Abdool-Karim of the University of KwaZulu-Natal is one South Africa's earliest scientists to work on HIV prevention, including vaccines. The *Castro-Hlongware* document characterizes Abdool-Karim's research as an "anti-human" activity promoted by "corporate forces." The document quotes sources spanning from the Bible to the World Health Organization. Most of the document centers on the toxic poisons that pharmaceutical companies sell as HIV treatments, indicting some of South Africa's leading AIDS scientists, including Glenda Gray and James McIntyre of the University of the Witwatersrand in Johannesburg, as co-conspirators in what would amount to racial genocide. Gray and McIntyre were singled out in the document because of their pioneering work in using antiretroviral medications for preventing mother-to-child HIV transmission. Along with Salim Abdool-Karim, Gray and McIntyre were included among the AIDS scientists on Mbeki's 2000 AIDS panel. Another main thrust of the *Castro-Hlongware's* document is that AIDS is nothing more than a cluster of old African diseases that stem from immune suppressing effects of malnutrition and poverty.

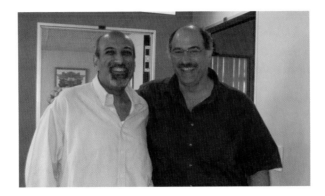

Photo 5.3 I have known Professor S. Salim Abdool Karim since 2001. Here I am visiting him at his researcher institute in Durban 2008

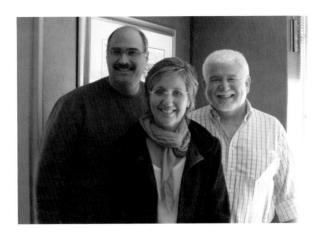

Photo 5.4 I met Professors Glenda Gray and James McIntyre in Johannesburg 2008

In summary, it would seem that South Africa was fertile ground for denialism to take root. The vicious policies of colonialism and Apartheid created an immense distrust of white authority and the West. The Apartheid regime had even worked on biological weapons to control the black population in the event of civil war. African liberation brought dreams of self-reliance – African solutions for African problems. Long standing cultural taboos on discussing sex and sexuality reinforced denial, secrecy, and stigma. An understandable focus on poverty and the shadow that it casts on all health problems detracted from any one disease. Finally, South Africa had a president who was suspicious and self-reliant on interpreting information, even some of the most complex of biological sciences. Denialists opportunistically seized the moment and hijacked the nation's health policy. Perhaps most bewildering of all is how the President of South Africa, who was devoted to finding African solutions and building self-sufficiency on the continent, came to believe a group of mostly American and European pseudoscientists and entrepreneurs over his own internationally acclaimed South African scientists.

The Durban Declaration

On the eve of the 2000 International AIDS conference, there was concern by the global scientific community that the world's attention to AIDS could be hampered by denialists given their prominent role in Mbeki's AIDS Panel. In an attempt to derail denialism in South Africa, over 5000 scientists and physicians, including Nobel Prize winners signed a brief statement designed to refute the claims of Duesberg and the other denialists. The statement was the first direct response to AIDS denialism by a group of international scientists. In July 2000, the journal *Nature* published what was soon called the Durban Declaration, which was titled "A Declaration by Scientists and Physicians Affirming HIV is the Cause of AIDS." The aim of the Durban Declaration was to debunk all of the major points of AIDS denialism, stating,

- The evidence that AIDS is caused by HIV-1 or HIV-2 is clear-cut, exhaustive and unambiguous, meeting the highest standards of science. The data fulfill exactly the same criteria as for other viral diseases, such as polio, measles and smallpox.
- Patients with acquired immune deficiency syndrome, regardless of where they live, are infected with HIV.
- If not treated, most people with HIV infection show signs of AIDS within five to ten years. HIV infection is identified in blood by detecting antibodies, gene sequences or viral isolation. These tests are as reliable as any used for detecting other virus infections.
- People who received HIV-contaminated blood or blood products develop AIDS, whereas those who received untainted or screened blood do not.
- Most children who develop AIDS are born to HIV-infected mothers. The higher the viral load in the mother, the greater the risk of the child becoming infected.
- In the laboratory, HIV infects the exact type of white blood cell (CD4 lymphocytes) that becomes depleted in people with AIDS.
- Drugs that block HIV replication in the test tube also reduce virus load in people and delay progression to AIDS. Where available, treatment has reduced AIDS mortality by more than 80%.
- Monkeys inoculated with cloned SIV DNA become infected and develop AIDS.[24]

At the International AIDS Conference, Mbeki maintained his view that poverty was a crisis in his country and that the cause of AIDS had not yet been determined, essentially ignoring the Durban Declaration. Mbeki stated:

> Therefore, being insufficiently educated, and therefore ill prepared to answer this question, I started to ask the question, expecting an answer from others – what is to be done, particularly about HIV-AIDS! One of the questions I have asked is – are safe sex, condoms and anti-retroviral drugs a sufficient response to the health catastrophe we face! I am pleased to inform you that some eminent scientists decided to respond to our humble request to use their expertise to provide us with answers to certain questions. Some of these have specialized on the issue of HIV-AIDS for many years and differed bitterly among themselves about various matters. Yet, they graciously agreed to join together to help us find answers to some outstanding questions. I thank them most sincerely for their positive response, inspired by a common resolve more effectively to confront the AIDS epidemic. They have agreed to report back by the end of this year having worked together, among other things, on the reliability of and the information communicated by our current HIV tests and the improvement of our disease surveillance system.[25]

As Michael Merson, former head of the Global AIDS Program at the World Health Organization, pointed out at the Durban AIDS conference that much of what Mbeki spoke of was true. Poverty is the cause of significant public health problems in his country including contributing to AIDS. However, Merson quickly reminds us that in the year 2000, there was no debate among credible scientists about the cause of AIDS. By calling for more research on whether HIV causes AIDS as if this was an unsettled question, the president of the country with the world's fastest growing AIDS epidemic placed denialism at the center of his national AIDS policy.

The saga of South Africa's Presidential AIDS Panel continued with 12 AIDS denialist members responding to the Durban Declaration, stating:

> Our objection to the Durban Declaration is factual and verifiable from data published in the early 1980s. We believe that World Health Organization (WHO) figures produced since then can be interpreted to say that AIDS first appeared and spread, not in Africa but in US urban clusters of mainly white, affluent, promiscuous homosexual men and drug addicts, and then spread, on a lesser scale, in Europe and Australasia but hardly at all in Asia. Disastrous epidemics due to heterosexual transmission of HIV were confidently predicted in general populations of developed countries but they never happened. AIDS has diminished in incidence and severity though it is continuing in female partners of bisexual men and some other communities engaging in or subjected to behaviors which carry high risks of infections, various assaults and misuse of drugs.[26]

The Durban Declaration and its subsequent response represent the only open exchange between international AIDS scientists and denialists. Although

Mbeki removed himself from the public "AIDS debate" following the 2000 International AIDS Conference, his policies, particularly those involving HIV treatments, have remained entrenched in denialism. Despite its greater wealth than any country in southern Africa, the Republic of South Africa has been the slowest to respond to AIDS, including failing to expand HIV testing and counseling programs at a scale in keeping with HIV prevalence, failing to offer HIV treatments to those infected and implementing programs to prevent mother-to-child HIV transmission. Today it is true that more South Africans are being treated for HIV, but the availability of treatment remains hampered by the government. Activists, particularly the Treatment Action Campaign, led by one of the world's most inspiring AIDS activist Zackie Achmat have taken legal action to increase treatment access. Their role remains central in the sustained efforts to provide HIV treatments.

AIDS Activism Meets Denialism

One of the more curious events in the history of AIDS has been the embracing of denialism by groups typically regarded as AIDS activists. For example, there is no shortage of performers, actors, and rock stars who have generously given their time to AIDS activism. Rock stars joining up with denialism, however, is rather bizarre. The popular rock group, the Foo Fighters, offers the most notable example. The Grammy Award winning band has been a vocal proponent of Christine Maggiore's denialist movement. The band aims to get the word out that HIV does not cause AIDS and had linked its web site to Christine Maggiore's *Alive and Well* web site. After having read Maggiore's book, band member Nate Mandel believes that "If you test positive, you are pretty much given a bleak outlook and told to take toxic drugs to possibly ward off new infections."[27]

Christine Maggiore herself had been an AIDS activist after she initially tested HIV positive. Later, having read about Duesberg and his associates, she came to question her own diagnosis and turned to denialism. Maggiore ultimately became perhaps the most influential denialism activist. An even earlier case of AIDS activism turned denialism is the Health Education AIDS Liaison (HEAL). HEAL was established in 1982 as a community organization to provide health information for people affected by AIDS, even before HIV testing became available. Today, HEAL is one of the most active denialist organizations, still centered on holistic treatments while defying HIV as the cause of AIDS. The organization sponsors events and holds member meetings in several cities with a considerable outreach effort. HEAL describes itself as having:

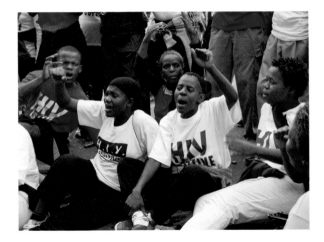

Photo 5.5 Treatment Action Campaign demonstration to bring HIV medications to South Africa, Cape Town 2003

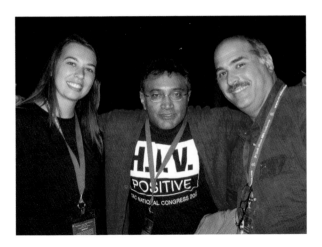

Photo 5.6 I have met South African AIDS activist Zackie Achmat several times. Here I am with him and fellow AIDS researcher Demetria Cain in Durban 2007

Come to discover that so far as 'AIDS' goes, we have been subject to the most heinous and genocidal fraud in medical history. And that to escape it, one must view not only AIDS, but all health and healthcare within an entirely different, life-affirming and self-empowering perspective. . . .Testing positive to HIV antibodies is even more misleading because all positive tests are likely to be false positives. The June '93 issue of the journal *Bio/Technology* published a review declaring the test to be scientifically invalid. Additionally, seropositive people do not necessarily develop AIDS and seronegative people may nonetheless develop AIDS.[28]

The vocal AIDS activist organization AIDS Coalition to Unleash Power (ACTUP) has been and remains the most visible AIDS political action group. Founded in the first days of the AIDS epidemic, ACTUP orchestrated dramatic demonstrations to raise awareness of the AIDS crisis, including holding funeral processions in Washington streets for people who had died of AIDS. The group effectively calls attention to suffering from AIDS and government inaction. ACTUP pressured the NIH to increase AIDS research, the Food and Drug Administration to accelerate drug approvals, and pharmaceutical companies to look for new treatments. In San Francisco, ACTUP/Golden Gate was one of the more effective organizations. In a strange turn of events, ACTUP/Golden Gate splintered and a fringe group emerged that refuted the established views of AIDS, including rejecting that HIV causes AIDS. The organization officially split in 2000, with Survive AIDS maintaining the original ACTUP mission and a new organization ACTUP/San Francisco advancing denialism. ACTUP/San Francisco stated that AIDS was constructed from an anti-gay agenda of the Reagan administration and that AZT and other HIV medications are poison. One irony to this whole episode is how a gay political organization could end up following the words of Duesberg, who has repeatedly spoken derogatorily about gays and the "gay lifestyle," including referring to gay men as "homos."[29] The death of prominent member David Pasquarelli in 2004 as well as other members of its leadership, including Michael Bellefountaine and Ronnie Bur, led to the disbanding of ACTUP/San Francisco.

Denialism activists also protest AIDS philanthropy and charities. Most notably, the Rethinking AIDS Society launched a public campaign against the Product Red initiative. Product Red was started by Irish musician and activist Bono to enlist businesses to donate profits to the Global Fund to Fight AIDS, Tuberculosis, and Malaria from the sale of items that are marketed with the Product Red logo (RED). One example is a clothing line marketed by The Gap stores where the Product (RED) logo is infused with affirming words, such as "INSPI(RED)" or "ADMI(RED)." The Rethinking AIDS group has produced materials and web sites that claim the RED initiative actually harms Africa, stating that Africa is "IGNO(RED)" by RED. They have even gone as far as to handout "IGNO(RED)" brochures at the entrance to RED fundraising events – claiming that the RED campaign stands for Racist-Elitist-Destructive. The warped perspective is well represented by journalist Neville Hodgkinson who said:

> Today, whether it is frightening the residents of a Cornish town with a cluster of purported infections, or causing the former head of South Africa's National AIDS Council (sic.) [Jacob Zuma] to apologize for having unprotected sex with an HIV-positive AIDS activist, or enabling U2 front-man Bono to edit an issue of the

independent newspaper dominated by impassioned accounts of Africa's HIV/AIDS plight, the virus that has held such sway in the popular mind for more than 20 years is still never long out of the news. It is now very big business: American Express, Motorola, Gap, Converse and Armani are among the corporate giants supporting Bono's RED campaign promoting special products to raise funds for AIDS in Africa.[30]

Denialist activism appears to be on the rise, bolstered by having its own rock band endorsers and its success in seeping into the popular press.

Political Ideologies

Given that much of HIV is about sex and socially marginalized groups, it is no surprise that religious and political extremism has intersected with denialism. Conservative religious organizations exerted considerable influence in the Reagan administration, fostering the AIDS denialist policies of the 1980s. The onset of AIDS at the time of the Reagan Republican Revolution provided the "religious right" with proof that God punishes sinners, such as homosexuals, drug users, and prostitutes. Today, there remains a clear connection between conservative political groups and at least some denialists.

Journalist Tom Bethell, for example, is the most well-recognized politically conservative commentator with an interest in intelligent design, Aneuploidy, and HIV/AIDS denialism. As a popular conservative writer and radio personality, Bethell reaches far more people with his denialist message than any esoteric journalist or AIDS pseudoscientist. Although he is not saying anything new about AIDS, by pointing to drugs and lifestyles as the cause of AIDS, Bethell has inspired a new generation of conservative denialists. Reaching a fringe medical audience, the online *Journal of Physicians and Surgeons* publishes papers that highlight the harms of abortion, the influence of immigration on the health-care system, alternative views on AIDS, and the "abnormalities" of the gay lifestyle. Presenting the impression of a mainstream medical journal, the *Journal of Physicians and Surgeons* has created a credible image for AIDS pseudoscience. Further solidifying their denialist stance, their affiliated organization, the Semmelweis Society, awarded Duesberg and Celia Farber their "Clean Hands" award in 2008 for whistle blowing on the truth about AIDS.

Conservative groups have also embraced AIDS pseudoscientist and Nessie expert Henry Bauer. For example, William F. Shughart of the University of Mississippi credits Henry Bauer with uncovering a "knowledge monopoly" erected by gay activists, drug companies, advisory panels of the federal Food and Drug Administration, academic researchers, and the governmental and non-governmental agencies that sponsor them. Bauer embraces the views of social conservatives when he claims that AIDS is the product of homosexual and drug using lifestyles as well as the genetics of Africans. The roots of Bauer's wacky ideas are easily traced to conservative ideologies, including his use of military HIV testing data to represent the US population.[31]

Social libertarianism, on the other hand, has appeared to confuse the right to free speech with scientific debate. From a free speech perspective, anyone would agree with the right to say that HIV does not cause AIDS, just as anyone can say the earth is flat and the Nazi Holocaust did not happen. Protecting free speech that masquerades as science potentially undermines the public trust and is therefore at issue because it poses the dilemma of protecting freedom for some at the expense of others. Nevertheless, social libertarians have bank rolled denialist projects, supported AIDS pseudoscience, and provided a home for denialist voices. Rebecca Culshaw, for example, made her denialism debut on the Lew Rockwell web site, which refers to itself as "anti-state, anti-war, pro-market" and the presidential campaign for libertarian Ron Paul had been briefed by leading AIDS conspiracy theorists.

Racism and Homophobia

Denialists have often turned the tables by claiming AIDS scientists are racist. Denialists say that AIDS science promotes the myth that Africans are hypersexual and primitive in their sexual behavior. Some denialists have claimed that by promoting the idea that sexual behavior spreads HIV we are blaming AIDS on the behavior of Africans, a falsehood that has helped fuel denialism in Africa. The racist overtones of baselessly declaring a genetic mechanism for testing HIV positive, such as proposed by Henry Bauer, is hardly subtle.[32] Canadian journalist David Crowe has made similar claims that fuel conspiracy theories about manufacturing HIV to control black populations.

The racism, sexism, and homophobia espoused by such rhetoric is quite telling about the political agendas of some denialists. A blatant effort exists to pit Africans and African-Americans against the white establishment, perhaps to fulfill self-proclaimed conspiracies. Homophobia thrives in denialism with claims that AIDS lifestyle choices, particularly drugs and sexual promiscuity, cause AIDS. The Perth Group, for example, has implicated repeated exposure to multiple sources of semen as immunosuppressive and causing AIDS. In an interview with the *Gay and Lesbian Times*, Duesberg repeated his basic premise that AIDS is caused by an unhealthy lifestyle and not HIV in overt homophobic terms:

You don't see it in the entire gay population...You're looking at a very small minority of the gay population who come to San Francisco or New York from the Midwest and so forth and they try to make it there as gay guys. There's peer pressure among them to have 20 or 30 dates in a weekend and wear a leather jacket – God knows what it is....Heterosexuals tend to get married or tend to go steady, so then the fun is over in this regard...What we call the 10-year latent period of HIV is a euphemism for the time it takes to cause irreversible damage by drug use.[33]

Duesberg's claim that gay lifestyles cause AIDS is consistent with conservative doctrines on homosexuality and has likely led to his warm reception by conservative groups. As noted by AIDS activist Martin Delaney, "In all his efforts to blame the victim for the disease, Duesberg has always overlooked the fact that there were plenty of gay men who died of AIDS who never had a history of either promiscuity or drug use. Whenever confronted with this information, Duesberg simply accused people of lying or being in denial."[34]

Bauer also has a history of homophobia. In a memoir, he wrote about his life in academic administration, Bauer wrote:

I have rather old-fashioned views: I regard homosexuality as an aberration or illness, not as an "equally valid life-style" or whatever the current euphemism may be. As with many aberrations and illnesses, I do not necessarily hold the individual responsible for being ill, and I do not believe that illness is criminal. Again as with many illnesses, I believe that some mixture of genetic or hereditary predisposition combines with environmental exposure to produce the actual condition....Thus I am not entirely in sympathy with gay student alliances, gay awareness festivals, or public forums to explain the validity of the gay life-style. I don't approve of proselytizing by gays; and I think it's very difficult to draw a line between free speech about civil rights for gays and the tendency for the life-style to be presented as something that it would be perfectly all right for anyone to choose.[35]

Beyond Duesberg and Bauer, homophobia is blatant in other denialist writings. Perhaps most notorious is Harvey Bialy who has used terms such as "faggot" and other derogatory references to homosexuality. John Lauritsen, an openly gay resident of Provincetown, Massachusetts and AIDS denialist wrote an essay titled *Has Provincetown Become Protease Town?* in which he states, "the 'magic of Provincetown' has become a magnet for gay men with diagnoses of 'AIDS' or 'HIV-positive'. For a decade now they have been arriving here – their medical records in hand, their various welfare benefits established, and their life insurance policy (if any) cashed in – to spend their final days in Provincetown." This apparent expression of internalized homophobia is not unique to denialism. What does represent a rather bizarre and unique feature of HIV/AIDS denialism is its repeated reference to AIDS scientists as Nazis.

The Nazi Thing

Denialists try to turn the tables on AIDS scientists by referring to them as Nazis. South African President Mbeki himself has compared AIDS scientists to the doctors of Nazi concentration camps. South African attorney Anthony Brink has made several allusions to Nazi Germany as a metaphor for the "poisoning" of South Africans with toxic drugs. Brink's Nazi imagery is particularly ironic given his association and employment by the German vitamin entrepreneur Matthias Rath. The cover of Brink's self-published book *Debating AZT* scripted AZT in an old German Gothic typeface that has an eerily familiar use in Nazi propaganda. The cover of his more recent self-published book uses a Nazi propaganda poster that depicts a young girl in a Hitler Youth uniform on which he added an AIDS-red ribbon on her lapel. In his self-published monograph *The Trouble with Nevirapine*, Brink mentions Nazi Germany more than a few times. In one case, he describes the pharmaceutical industry as promoting AZT in a lie on a "Nazi scale." In the same document, he refers to AIDS activist Zackie Achmat by saying "Like the Third Reich, however, we find that the TAC [Treatment Action Campaign] is led by a prodigiously energetic but ignorant buffoon, driven by an irrepressible sense of public purpose." And in a third reference Brink describes The President of the International AIDS Society Mark Weinberg as having his "back pocket" stuffed from overseeing nevirapine clinical trials. Brink describes his reaction to hearing Wainberg's address at the International AIDS Conference in this way:

> I watched this guy with his Colgate smile glad-handing several dazzled women at a lunch table at Durban's AIDS Conference in 2000 a couple of paces from where I sat. The International AIDS hero. And I couldn't help recalling that timeless summation of Eichman(sic): "The banality of evil."[36]

I spoke with Anthony Brink while he was, ironically enough, visiting Berlin and asked him about his reference to Aldolf Eichmann, who was responsible for the mass deportation of Jews to extermination camps in Nazi Germany. Brink laughed and asked me if I thought he was a Nazi? His words, not mine.

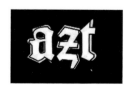

Displays 5.3 Adaptation of Anthony Brink's book cover Debating azt: Mbeki and the AIDS drug controversy, self published by Anthony Brink. This adaptation shows the type face used that alludes to Nazism in reference to AZT

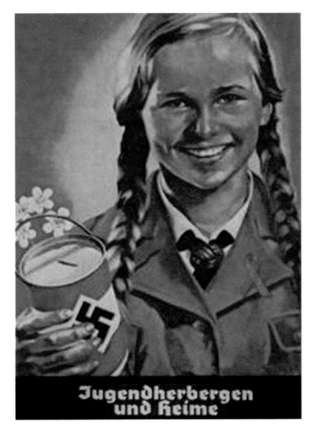

Displays 5.4 Adaptation of Anthony Brink's book cover Just say yes, Mr. President: Mbeki and AIDS self published by Anthony Brink. This adaptation shows the use of a classic Nazi propaganda poster with an AIDS red ribbon digitally pasted to the lapel. The book cover also removed the German text and replaced it with the book title

Denialists use Nazi images and references to dramatize what they see as the poisoning of societies with antiretrovirals. They talk about the inhumane experimentation and coercion that is used to force drugs on the innocent, particularly children with AIDS, drawing the comparison of AIDS scientists with Nazi doctors. The great irony of the denialists' Nazi allusions to AIDS scientists, of course, is that they base their argument on the views of a group of German men born during the years of Nazism while making Nazi references to AIDS scientists, who are often Jews.

AIDS Denialism in the Courtroom

Denialists have at times launched law suits against individuals and organizations that distribute and administer antiretroviral therapies. For example, South African attorney Brink has sued the Treatment Action Campaign for their efforts to bring antiretrovirals to South Africa. These law suits have been a key element in slowing treatments access in that country. In another example, The Alberta Reappraising AIDS Society awarded its 2004 SARAH Award to San Francisco attorney David Steele for his suing the pharmaceutical company GlaxoSmithKlein, in which he claimed that administering AZT to a young boy who was exposed to HIV in a medical needle stick accident recklessly put the child at risk for developing cancer. AZT is widely known to avert HIV transmission in such cases when administered within hours of HIV exposure and the drug is now used routinely with rape victims and medical exposure accidents in what is called post-exposure prophylaxis. It should be expected that denialists will continue to move their cause to the courts given the litigiousness of suspicious thinkers, paranoid personalities, and conspiracy theorists.

Denialism is also creeping into the criminal courts. With AIDS pseudoscience available as evidence and the false sense of legitimacy offered by a Presidential AIDS Advisory Panel, there is growing use of denialism as a criminal defense. The most illustrative case is that of Andre Parenzee, an HIV-positive Australian man who had sex with a number of women without disclosing his HIV status. In January of 2006, the 36-year-old Parenzee was convicted on three counts of endangering the life of a woman he had infected with HIV. Parenzee appealed his conviction, arguing that a judge had failed to take into account the different "streams of scientific thought about the cause of AIDS." His defense attorney called prominent denialists on his behalf, including Elani Papadopulos-Eleopulos who the judge later rejected as an AIDS expert. The judge did accept the testimony of established AIDS scientists who refuted the defense's arguments that HIV does not exist and could not be sexually transmitted. Parenzee's original conviction was upheld. Journalist David Crowe took up a collection to continue the legal fight for Parenzee. Crowe stated "These HIV positive people being thrown in jail have almost always had consensual sex with their partners. Mostly they are heterosexual men, like Andre Parenzee, but sometimes they are homosexual men, or heterosexual women. Consent by their partners is decreed to be void based on the legal system's complete and utter ingestion of the HIV=AIDS=Death dogma."[37]

Another legal case championed by denialists is that of Trevis Smith, a Canadian football player who had not informed his girlfriend about his HIV positive status. The woman became infected with HIV and Smith had unprotected sex with two other women, exposing them to the virus when he knew he was infected. Smith received 5-1/2 years in prison. Another case concerned Canadian businessman Carl Leone who had as many as 20 sex partners. In another case, Johnson Aziga was charged with first-degree murder, because three of his sex partners were found HIV-positive and subsequently died of

AIDS. In all three cases, denialists complained that the defendants were treated unfairly because they did not harm anyone, because of course HIV does not cause AIDS.

Body Bags

A Stop AIDS Chicago activist I once knew posed the question, "what will it take for politicians and people in power to realize what is going on with AIDS? Does it take body bags?" As the AIDS death toll has risen, the demand for attention to AIDS has also grown. Unfortunately, history has shown that body bags do not persuade politicians to act or inspire sound AIDS policy.

A blatant example that I discussed earlier is the US federal ban on needle exchange programs. Scientists reached consensus in the early 1990s that needle exchange programs effectively prevent HIV infections at no harm to society while there is no evidence that abstinence only prevention programs effectively prevent pregnancy or sexually transmitted infections. Still, the US federal ban on providing clean needles and syringes for HIV prevention has remained in place. US federal laws also require abstinence-based education in government sponsored HIV/AIDS prevention programs. There is also no evidence for any public health security value in restricting US immigration based on HIV status, but the provision has until recently remained in place. Everyone knows that prison inmates engage in sex while they risk all sorts of infections by using objects such as the fingers of latex gloves as makeshift condoms. Still condoms remain contraband in state and federal prisons. The South African Minister of Health has retained Roberto Giraldo as a key policy advisor, recommending the use of African potatoes, beetroot, garlic, and olive oil for treating AIDS while blocking access to antiretroviral therapies. In South Africa, babies of HIV infected mothers are still being born with HIV, whereas universal testing and treatment programs in neighboring countries such as Botswana have plummeted the number of HIV infected babies to nearly zero. Sadly, numbers of AIDS cases and AIDS deaths have typically not altered AIDS policies and there is no reason to suspect they will as long as denialism persists. It seems then that our greatest hope is to find a way out of denialism, or at least to expose it for what it is.

Getting Out of Denial 6

You can move a person out of denial by deliberately provoking them to anger. Hold up the future (sympathetically) so they cannot avoid or deny it. Tell them that it is not fair. Show anger yourself.
Elisabeth Kübler-Ross

Having immersed myself in the world of denialism, upon reflection I think it is best summed up as resembling a beehive. At first glance, denialism appears to be a chaotic swam of senseless and haphazard activity. But all of that random activity is really deceptive. Closer inspection reveals a highly organized social structure of leaders and drones, all sharing the common purpose of protecting the hive. I would not go as far as to say that denialism is as organized as a beehive, but it is also a mistake to think that denialism is a chaotic swam. What at first may appear to be a few crackpots and deranged scientists exploiting AIDS for some self-indulging gratification turns out to be a far more complex social and psychological phenomenon. And of course, sticking your hand in the hive will mean you will surely be stung.

What then is the social order of denialism? I see denialism as a whole best characterized as a three-tiered pyramid scheme. The top tier has been the focus of this book, occupied by those denialists who write literature to propagate AIDS myths. Their words are the most persuasive and provide the very basis for the denialist movement. The second tier is composed of those suspicious minded persons who gravitate toward conspiracy theories and pretty much anything that is anti-establishment. The individuals in this tier also propagate denialism because they contribute to discussions, list-serves, blogs, and whatever opportunities arise to express denialist beliefs. The third and largest tier of denialism is the least visible but it is also the most concerning. These people are most likely affected by AIDS, often having tested positive themselves or having a loved one who has tested HIV positive. These are often people who doubt their health care providers and already mistrust the health care system. Ultimately, people affected by AIDS risk the greatest harm from denialism.

Denialism in all of its forms does the most harm to those who are its object, in this case people living with HIV/AIDS. All denialists can make for entertaining television and radio talk show programming. But Holocaust deniers inspire anti-Semitism, embolden neo-Nazis, instigate hate crimes, and even provide a rationale for heads of state to refute the legitimacy of Israel, as did Iranian President Mahmūd Ahmadīnezhādor in 2006 when he organized a conference to discuss whether the Holocaust had ever occurred. The greatest harm done by Holocaust deniers is to the Holocaust survivors. In the same way, it is the people who are convinced by denialists to refuse cancer chemotherapy and to instead take mega-doses of vitamins are the ones harmed by cancer denialism. And yet again, those most harmed by HIV/AIDS denialism are those who are infected with the virus. There are now countless HIV infected people who have avoided getting tested for HIV, rejected their HIV positive test results, ignored safer sex practices, failed to disclose their HIV status to sex partners, and refused HIV treatments for themselves and their children because they have believed denialists. Health decisions that are disinformed by denialist rhetoric are why we must care about denialism.

In and Out of Denialism

Having read a great deal of what the denialists have to say and having communicated at length with several of them myself, I am left to question how much any of these people actually care about AIDS and those affected by the disease. Denialists are often as obsessed with toxins causing cancer as they are with HIV not causing AIDS. These are the same people who are no more willing to accept chemotherapy for treating cancer than they are willing to accept anti-HIV medications. Interestingly, these same denialists implicate the National Institutes of Health, Big Pharma, etc. in both cancer and AIDS conspiracies. They also sell the same vitamins and potions for both cancer and AIDS. What denialists do apparently care about is the argument itself. It is the debate that seems to drive their interest in AIDS, not the other way around. None of the major figures in denialism has ever worked with HIV in the laboratory and none have worked with people infected with HIV. Some, including South Africa's president, have gone as far as to say that they have never even known a person who has died of AIDS, despite people close to them, sometimes even their children, having died of AIDS. This lack of sensitivity to the human side of AIDS brings me to conclude that denialism is nothing more than a callous stream of pontification devoid of any socially redeeming value.

In some cases HIV positive parents, such as Kathleen Tysob of Eugene, Oregon and Canadian Sophie Brassard, have lost custody of their children for not providing them with HIV treatments after having been persuaded by the denialists. In other cases, such as Noreen Martin of South Carolina, people turn to holistic approaches to healing themselves, an individual choice that surely would be respectable if not for proselytizing to others. There are now web sites dedicated to people living with HIV/AIDS who provide testimonials regarding their discovery of denialism. For example, the web sites for Living without HIV Drugs, Alive and Well, and even the personal web site of University of Miami Biochemistry Professor Rudolf Werner lists the stories of people who tested HIV positive and chose to forego antiretroviral therapies. All of these people share in common their having gotten sicker when they were taking anti-HIV medications and then suddenly experiencing improved health when they stopped taking the drugs. Some say they have stopped for years. Their stories are all similar to Christine Maggiore's and offer a glistening lure to people in search of a cure.

I spoke with one man who posted his story on the Living without HIV Drugs web site about his decision to refuse treatments. He was definitely not in denial about his HIV status nor did he proselytize others to stop their treatment. He simply chose a path of natural remedies as his approach to managing his HIV infection. He had a partner who had taken HIV treatments and died of AIDS. He did not question the fact that HIV diminishes the immune system. He also did not question whether HIV causes AIDS. However, he did not feel the medications to treat HIV were the right thing for him personally. I found him genuine and caring, and he was not interested in persuading others to do what he had found right for himself. I believe that his views were also misrepresented by including them on the Living without HIV Drugs web site. Surely he was living without taking the medications, but the aims of the web site clearly say why they share these stories: "We want to share our stories with you, in hopes that they can be an inspiration and provide you with the hope that you, too, can live without HIV drugs and their very serious and damaging side effects. Keep in mind that the HIV medications that you may be taking now (or will probably be pressured into taking if you are newly diagnosed as HIV-Positive) can be, and often are more dangerous than the HIV."[1]

There are also as many postings online of people who say they were lured into denialism, later realizing that they were getting sicker and in need of treatment. These stories also share some common characteristics including being coaxed into denialism and refusing treatment only to become quite ill and propelled back into reality. The following examples of people who were in and then out of denialism illustrate these themes:

I can testify that it isn't just newly diagnosed or vulnerable people who are likely to buy the denialist message. Well-educated on the subject and 10 years into the illness, I started reading the denialist arguments and they are very alluring. I stopped meds…became sick for the first time. I had an AIDS denialist doctor who told me to just stay off the meds even though my T-cells were in steady decline and I was beginning to opportunistic infections. When pressed, he admitted that it was all an "experiment" for him. I'm finally back on meds and doing well and VERY thankful for them, and thankful I didn't get worse than I did.

I was compelled by denialist thinking in the 90s. As an economist, their "follow the money" arguments made sense. In 2003 I left myself vulnerable for AIDS related Lymphoma because I was afraid yes, AFRAID to start HIV meds because of very compelling arguments by Peter Duesberg, Christine Maggiore & others… Four years on ATRIPLA [a 3-drug combination antiretroviral medication] – thankfully – after severe illness (following denialist recommendations) opened my eyes. On HIV meds, I have never felt better.[2]

One of the more famous cases of a person who moved into and out of denialism is the Zambian AIDS activist Wistone Zulu. His story is remarkably similar to those who report their initial attraction to denialism. Zulu had come to doubt whether HIV causes AIDS. As a well known activist in southern Africa, he was invited to serve on South Africa's now infamous 2000 Presidential AIDS panel. Zulu talks about how he saw the questions being raised about AIDS by the "dissidents" on the presidential AIDS panel as a way out of his HIV infection. He had always believed in questioning medicine and seeking alternative opinions. But now he believes that is where he went wrong, by listening to sources that appeared credible because of their credentials and accepting their word. He describes his seduction into denialism like this:

Amongst those that said HIV does not cause AIDS was Kary Mullis, the man who invented polymerase chain re-action – one of the technologies used to measure viral load. He went on to win the Nobel Prize for that. Perhaps the most well known dissident is Peter Duesberg, who until he espoused his dissident views was considered one of the top scientists in the USA. He, among other things, discovered oncogenes thought to be the cause of some cancers. He was a member of the American Academy of Scientists and used to receive thousands of dollars from the government for his research. Last but not least there is David Rasnick who is a recognized expert on protease inhibiters. There were also a number of others with impressive scientific and medical backgrounds who somehow felt the science did not add up. In other words, for me it was very hard to tell who was really in the know. What mattered to me as person living with HIV was to be told that HIV did not cause AIDS. That was nice. Of course, it was like printing money when the economy is not doing well. Or pissing in your pants when the weather is too cold. Comforting for a while but disastrous in the long run.[3]

Zulu had fallen ill from fungal infections and was so fatigued and that he could not walk. He then says he came to realize that "denialism was a lie." He reversed his decision and sought treatment. His health improved and he has remained on HIV treatments, becoming one of southern Africa's most vocal activists against denialism.

Why Denialism Will Not Go Away

One of the themes I have tried to communicate in this book is that denialism is self-perpetuating. It has therefore been a mistake of the past to ignore denialists in the hope that they will simply go away. If anything, denialism is becoming more prominent. Since 2006, several new denialist web sites have appeared, blogs have emerged, articles have appeared in the mainstream press, and books have been published. Mind you these new books say nothing new, but their increased presence is worrisome.

In just one year, between 2007 and 2008, The Rethinking AIDS Society has reorganized and spruced up its web site with David Crowe as the new president of the society. Rethinking AIDS has also gained a new media-public relations person and has launched a disinformation campaign against the Product (RED) initiative to provide HIV treatments in Africa. AIDS Rethinkers have also started to produce pod-casts and have appeared in several albeit irregular and off-beat radio talk shows. Also in the past year Peter Duesberg has experienced his own renaissance, with a full feature article in *Discover* magazine and a whistle blowers award from the Semmelweis Society, which he shared with Celia Farber.

Also in just the past year the President of South Africa Thabo Mbeki fired his progressive Deputy Health Minister who fell out of line with South Africa's denialist policies. We also learned from an acclaimed biography of President Mbeki that he remains entrenched in denialism. The past year has also given us another African head of state, President Yahya Jammeh of Gambia, who claims that he can personally cure people of AIDS. The past year also found the US presidential campaign embroiled in controversy over Barack Obama's former minister espousing his beliefs that HIV was developed by the government as a genocidal weapon against the African American community. The year also saw the persistence of denialist US policies from mandating abstinence based prevention programming, to banning needle exchange funding to restricting the entry of visitors with HIV/AIDS.

Given these recent events and the ever growing presence of denialism on the Internet, we should not expect denialism to go away. Although the first generation of denialists, and their AIDS scientist counter parts for that matter, are not getting any younger, it would be foolish to believe that the death of the most visible denialists would lead to a demise of the denialist movement. Denialism, like any other corpus, lives on. There is also a second generation of denialists, including pseudoscientists, fringe academics, and journalists who all seem amply ready to carry the denialism touch. If anything, we should expect the deaths of the old guard to create a new class of denialist – martyrs. Indeed, when denialists are suspected to have died of AIDS their deaths become yet another spoke in the wheel of denialism.

When Denialists Die

Everybody dies eventually. But when a denialist is suspected to have died from AIDS it receives unique attention. On the one hand, anti-denialists seize the moment, using the deaths of denialists to make the point that these people have died earlier than they should have from a treatable disease. On the flipside, denialists are quick to respond that their comrades died of anything other than AIDS. One particularly vivid example was when prominent denialist activist of ACTUP San Francisco David Pasquarelli died in 2004 at age 37. It was widely held that he developed several HIV-related illnesses and succumbed to AIDS. However, because he also had served a jail term for activist-related charges, Christine Maggiore quickly claimed that the conditions that Pasquarelli encountered in jail killed him, not AIDS. In a response to Pasquarelli's death, Maggiore wrote the following rationalization:

> Dave became ill after spending almost three months in jail without decent food, proper rest, and fearing for his life in almost every moment. He went in as a thin but healthy vegetarian who rode his bike all over the hills of San Francisco and as someone with food allergies and a childhood history of respiratory issues. He came out of jail malnourished, dehydrated, physically ill and emotionally exhausted. . . . While incarcerated, Dave had to live on a prison diet which is very low in quality and nutritional content, high in sugar and empty carbohydrates and he was prohibited from taking vitamins. He lived in a cell with an exhaust vent connected to the laundry room where inmates' uniforms were washed in toxic chemical detergents. Dave told me he would often wake up in the morning covered with a thin layer of orange fuzz that came from machines drying the inmates uniforms. He said they used floor stripper for laundry detergent when they ran out of soap. He also told me he was given unidentified immunizations without his consent. After Dave was released on bail, he realized that the only way to avoid trial and the possibility of returning to jail was to be sick. Being ill became a strategy and this situation turned into a medical nightmare in many ways including stints at Saint Mary's hospital where he could stay at no cost but received less than attentive care. For example, after complaining that an IV drip in his hand hurt, the shunt was

finally removed and a staff infection was noted (a common infection in HIV negatives in hospital settings), but by this time, the staff infection had gone systemic affecting his internal organs.[4]

Needless to say, many people endure much harsher jail sentences of longer duration than did Pasquarelli and they do not die of immune system failure. People develop infections but they do not typically become systemic in the absence of severely depressed immunity. Maggiore makes the important point that it may be unfair to draw conclusions on a person's cause of death in the absence of medical records and factual accounts. Nevertheless, the inability to penetrate denialist beliefs is apparent in the twists and turns used to spin these deaths. Being without satisfying relationships, unemployment, in financial trouble, depression, loss of friends and lovers, are all attributed causes for immune system decline and ultimately death of denialists. In the eyes of denialists, virtually anything could have killed these young people except for AIDS.

The anti-denialist web site aidstruth.org has created a memorial for when denialists die. In most cases, it is apparent that they had died of AIDS. Of course, even with treatment many or even all of these people would have died anyway. However, the evidence is overwhelming that if they had been treated their HIV infection would have slowed and AIDS may have been delayed. A few of the more notable examples of how denialists have spun the deaths of fellow denialists are presented here, as they were extracted from aidstruth.org:[5]

Robert Johnston a co-founder of HEAL Toronto and a co-author of the self-described a "rebuttal" of the Durban Declaration, where he wrote "Robert Johnston is a co-founder of HEAL Toronto, and has been HIV-positive since 1985 yet has suffered no unusual illness since that time. He attributes his good health to not taking any anti-HIV medications and to not believing that his positive antibody test has much significance."Johnston died in 2003. David Crowe wrote that he died of "liver failure completely unrelated to AIDS."

Raphael Lombardo was a gay man who believed Peter Duesberg's claims that HIV was harmless. Lombardo wrote to Duesberg on May 30, 1995, noting that he had never used any recreational drugs or pharmaceuticals and was not sick, despite testing HIV positive. Duesberg published the entire letter in his book "Inventing the AIDS Virus" and wrote of Lombardo: "His letter proves that true science does not depend on institutional authority." Raphael Lombardo died of AIDS a little over a year later, on June 11, 1996. When asked about Lombardo's death, Duesberg wrote, "In hindsight, I think his letter was almost too good to be true. I am afraid now, he described the man he wanted to be [e.g. that he did not use recreational drugs] and his Italian family expected him to be, but not the one he really was. I think he died from Kaposi's."

Peter Mokaba a senior politician in South Africa's African National Congress Party and a prominent HIV/AIDS denialist, died in 2002 at the age of 43 from AIDS-related pneumonia after a "long illness." He denied that he had AIDS and rejected antiviral drugs as poison. His death is often noted because of his close association with President Mbeki who claims to have never known anyone who has died of AIDS.

Marietta Ndziba was used by the vitamin entrepreneur Matthias Rath to market multivitamins as an alternative to antiretroviral treatment. In a pamphlet distributed in Cape Town, South Africa in September 2005, she was quoted saying that her CD4 count rose from 365 to 841 due to Rath's vitamins. She implied that these vitamins treated boils on her arm, her grey skin, diarrhea and vomiting. She said, "I just thank God that he brings vitamins here to South Africa to help our lives." According to the South African AIDS activist organization Treatment Action Campaign, Ndziba never took antiretrovirals. She died in about October 2005. One family member reportedly claimed that she died of a stress headache.

AIDS Realism

AIDS realism is best achieved through an objective and critically minded look at the AIDS science. But here lies the problem. Understanding the science as it is published in the scientific literature requires technical knowledge in a variety of complicated sciences, everything from biochemistry to virology. No one human being can possibly understand it all. As a psychologist, I have been trained to understand AIDS behavioral science. How foolish I would be to think that I could fully grasp the fundamentals of protein synthesis, reverse transcription, molecular bonding dynamics, genetic mutations, and who knows what else is involved in the biology of HIV infection. How then can I be so certain that HIV causes AIDS? As I have said several times in this book, it is a matter of trust. I trust the tens of thousands of research studies conducted by the thousands of scientists across the globe who also conclude that HIV causes AIDS. I also trust the structural engineers who say that the World Trade Center could not have gone down by a controlled demolition. I also trust the Holocaust survivors who say they were in Auschwitz. I also trust that the world is not flat, despite the way that it looks to me from 33,000 feet above.

AIDS realism requires that we trust true experts and scientists who know more than we do to decipher the technical details. It is all about trust. And this is where it gets tricky. How can I be so sure that I am not being duped by Big Pharma, etc? What is my trust based on? My trust is grounded in three principles: credibility, contemporaneousness, and common sense.

Credibility

Earlier I discussed peer review for all its strengths and weaknesses. Still peer review is the best gage we have for assuring scientific authenticity. It used to be more difficult to know whether a scientist is established in the peer reviewed research literature. It is easier today to examine the messenger because of the Internet. Anyone can search the National Library of Medicine web site, http://www.ncbi.nlm.nih.gov, to find the work that any scientist has published in the peer-reviewed research literature. Let us say I search in the PubMed database for the name David Rasnick, who is often described as a prominent American biochemist. I will find 32 entries, most concerning Aneuploidy and some denote that they are correspondences or letters to editors, which are not peer reviewed. I can also see that Rasnick has as claimed by denialists, published on protease inhibitors, a key type of drug used in treating HIV. But Rasnick's work was with rats, not humans and for arthritis, not HIV. It is also easy to search the National Institutes of Health grants database, http://crisp.cit.nih.gov/crisp/c. Rasnick is not to be found in this data base. Looking further on the Internet, we can see that denialists claim that there is a censorship against AIDS dissidents, so perhaps Rasnick has been excluded from peer reviewed publication and NIH grants. How then does one achieve prominence in biochemistry while also being censored by the entire field of biochemistry? Researching denialists will ultimately lead to these same inherent contradictions between being an expert on the one hand and not having evidence whatsoever of expertise in HIV or AIDS.

   With the notable exception of Peter Duesberg, there are no denialists who have the credibility that comes with passing through the filters of peer review. That is what makes Duesberg such an anomaly. It is his history of scholarship and science that brought him to be taken seriously by the scientific community. But Duesberg's current standing confuses credentials with credibility.

Contemporaneousness

Defined as being current or of the present, science should be evaluated in light of its contemporaneousness. Today, AIDS science moves at a faster pace than any other area of medical research, with the possible exception of cancer. To understand AIDS one should not have to look back further than the past few years. For the consumer-reader, if a scientific article was published before 2000, I would say it can be considered dated, perhaps even ignored. Books published since 2000 should also be inspected for the age of their sources. Any writing in the area of AIDS that relies on sources from the 1980s should be suspect. Of the more than 116,000 scientific articles listed in the PubMed database concerning the HIV disease process, or HIV pathogenesis, over 31,000 have been published in the past 5 years. AIDS scientists are basing their conclusion that HIV causes AIDS on these current studies and these same researchers conclude that HIV treatments slow the progression of HIV to AIDS.

Common Sense

Think about it. Think about the gay men who never used drugs, who had been perfectly healthy and died of AIDS before there were antiretroviral medications. Suggesting that all gay men who have died of AIDS had used drugs, as Duesberg has claimed, reveals a stereotypic view of the gay community that can be considered nothing less than homophobic. Think about the fact that most people who test HIV positive do so late in the course of their HIV infection, many only after they had developed AIDS. Many of the people I have known who have tested HIV positive were indeed prompted to get tested because they became ill, including partners of injection drug users who themselves had never used drugs. How is it possible to believe that HIV treatments caused AIDS in these people? Think of the countless women with AIDS who have been infected with HIV by bisexual men; women who have not used drugs and who were ill before they get tested. Think about Africa. Is there any rationality in saying that AIDS is caused by poverty when some of the most impoverished countries in the world have no AIDS while southern Africa's richest country has among the largest AIDS problems? Blaming AIDS on drug abuse, HIV treatments, and poverty is an affront to every person living with this disease. Denialism is perhaps most offensive because it is an insult to our most basic common sense.

Critical Thinking – The Denialism Antidote

Unlike the scientific literature, denialist rhetoric is aimed at the general public. Denialist rhetoric can be quite convincing and alluring to almost anyone diagnosed with HIV. Delving into the science of AIDS on the Internet has become easier and sciences easily confused with pseudoscience. AIDS realism requires us to be at once open minded to find the newest in research and critical thinking to avoid being duped by the denialists. Below are some guidelines for using and interpreting medical and scientific findings reported on the Internet and in the media.[6]

Avoid Falling into Single Study Fallacies

No one research finding ever proves anything. Even the most compelling research studies require further analysis and independent replication before scientists themselves draw firm conclusions. One red flag is raised when a summary of research extracts a single sentence from a study to make the case for an argument. It is likely that the study finding is being exploited for the sake of denialism.

Consider the Source

Credibility of where the article is reported as well as the researchers themselves must be weighed when you hear about new research. As I discussed, credibility is built on reputations and trust, both of which can be very difficult to assess. Doing some investigative digging in credible places, like PubMed, can help. Information found on the Internet can be evaluated with the help of watchdog groups such as quackwatch.com. Red flags for Internet web sites include being based on old sources, especially dating back to the 1980s, not having a time stamp of their own with dates and updates, having dead-end links, and not providing contact information.

More Technical Does Not Mean More Credible

Reporters of sound medical science strive to simplify information whereas denialists and pseudoscientists create confusion through over-complexity. Lots of graphs and mathematical formulas can be a warning sign that the intent is to dazzle rather than inform.

If It Is too Good to Be True, It Probably Isn't

This old adage has been revitalized in the information age. Claims for cures and remarkable breakthroughs travel fast online. Trust your instincts and ask a friend for their opinion. Do not purchase a medical treatment without digging deeper to learn more about it.

Take It Up with Your Doctor

Finding new information about a medical condition is exciting and searching for information online can be empowering. Most doctors appreciate when their patients bring them new information to discuss. Asking your doctor if something new could work for you can help integrate each piece of care into the big picture. If you feel that your doctor does not listen to you when you bring him or her new information, or does not approach such information with an open mind, find a new doctor.

Be a Skeptic Not a Cynic

Not everyone is a doctor or scientist. When you find new medical information in a magazine or on the Internet, examine it with a keen eye of caution. Ask others what they think of the information. Look for independent sources that can confirm what you have found.

Be a Dissident, Not a Denialist

Remember, science has made great advances when pushed by outside thinkers. Being a dissident means listening to all sides and weighing the evidence. When a different view seems reasonable, entertain it. Challenge it. And when the credible evidence is overwhelming, accept it. The AIDS dissidents who have maintained their credibility are those who accepted the evidence that HIV causes AIDS and moved on to make new contributions. Those who refused to move on are stuck in denialism.

Anti-denialism

In keeping with one of nature's basic laws, for every action there is an equal and opposite reaction. The world of denialism is therefore met with the anti-denialist movement. Anti-denialists are, for the most part, the very same AIDS scientists, journalists, and activists who have been the target of the denialists themselves. The *Durban Declaration* that was published in 2000 (Chapter 5) was the first major effort by scientists to counter denialism. Coming off of the International AIDS Conference in Durban South Africa, especially after President Mbeki embraced the denialists, AIDS scientists have since published editorials in major newspapers and have written extensive commentaries and correction pieces on denialism and AIDS pseudoscience. The *Durban Declaration* marked a major shift among AIDS scientists who had ignored denialism hoping it would simply go away. Failing to respond to denialists became impossible, especially once they were embraced by South Africa's President.

Significant efforts to combat denialism have come from AIDS activists, scientists, and journalists. Martin Delaney, a San Francisco AIDS activist, has countered AIDS misinformation and disinformation through his work as Director of Project Inform, a leading AIDS information and education organization. Among the most visible anti-denialists are John Moore, an AIDS scientist at Cornell University, Mark Wainberg a leading clinical AIDS researcher at McGill University, and Jeanne Bergman, at The Center for HIV Law and Policy in New York City. They have published pieces to raise awareness of denialism in several high profile outlets, including the *New York*

Times, and regularly engage in counter arguments on Internet blogs and various web sites. In South Africa, the Treatment Action Campaign's Nathan Geffen and University of Cape Town Professor Nicoli Nattrass have been at the forefront of refuting denialism in their country.

One of the more colorful examples of anti-denialists responding to denialism came when a group of scientists and activists documented more than 50 fundamental errors in Celia Farber's 2006 article "Out of Control" published in *Harper's* magazine. Like the need to respond to Mbeki's AIDS panel with the *Durban Declaration*, the response to Farber was necessitated by the visibility that *Harpers* magazine brought to denialism. A group of AIDS scientists, journalists, and activists started aidstruth.org which defines its mission around the need to respond to Farber's *Harper's* article, stating "In March 2006, after *Harper's* magazine published a feature article by AIDS denialist Celia Farber, a number of scientists and activists joined together to create a web site for the purpose of countering AIDS denialist misinformation and debunking denialist myths, while providing truthful information about HIV and AIDS. The result is the aidstruth.org web site."[7] Because most of denialism is spread via the Internet, anti-denialists have established a considerable presence online. In this sense, anti-denialism is meeting denialism on its own turf.

Another significant anti-denialism presence online has been launched by one of the most credible and widely used sources for AIDS information, thebody. com, which has rapidly responded to denialism with commentaries and open forums. AIDS scientists have also become more active in responding to denialist claims on the Internet directly by writing letters to editors, university administrators, and others who could be misled into thinking denialist claims are legitimate dissidents.

Defeating Denialism

We have learned the hard way that denialism will not be defeated by ignoring it. Denialism will also not be defeated in a debate. Educating people about the basic truths of AIDS is of course essential to defeating denialism, but it would seem that education alone will not be enough. The mistrust of science and medicine behind denialism will not be penetrated by education campaigns and easy-to-understand brochures. For the part of the AIDS scientists, we must become better at communicating with people other than our fellow scientists. We also have to stop making predictions about the future that only undermine our credibility when they do not pan out. Legitimate dissidents in AIDS science should also have greater visibility. It helps the science when the public sees that there are legitimate disagreements among scientists. Having a more transparent scientific process will help dispel myths that reduce scientists to a monolithic orthodoxy. Public trust in science will also benefit from explanations of peer review, for all of its strengths and shortcomings. Making science and medicine more accessible to the public will help people distinguish between real science and that which masquerades as science.

Trust is also established when doctors, nurses, and other health care providers listen to their patients. Being open to complimentary treatments can make the difference in keeping patients on their course of treatment. Patients should be informed of what to expect in terms of side-effects with solutions in hand for managing them when they do occur. I have been struck by how many people turn to alternative remedies because they felt their doctor did not listen to their needs or concerns. There is no harm in a person taking their HIV treatments with blueberry juice, but telling them that they are crazy to think their blueberry juice will clean their body of toxic poisons will only serve to alienate some patients while infuriating others. Patients who trust their providers have fewer reasons to turn to denialism.

Journalists also play a critical role in defeating denialism. Journalists cannot rely solely on scientific credentials for authenticity and unfortunately tenure makes it impossible to know whether scientists are credible simply because they hold a professorship at an esteemed university. Journalism does a disservice to the public when denialists and pseudoscientists are elevated to legitimacy simply because they have the stature of an emeritus or professorship or whatever. It should matter when a professor who espouses that HIV is a harmless passenger virus also claims that there is no genetic basis for any cancers, or when a Nobel Laureate who says that HIV may not even exist also says that he has been abducted by aliens, or when a Professor Emeritus claims he has found the proof that HIV does not cause AIDS also says that he believes in big green monsters lurking beneath Scottish waters. None of these facts are hidden and they should not be ignored when journalists engage in real fact finding.

Ultimately, everyone who cares about AIDS and those who are affected by this scourge has a responsibility to defeat denialism. It's easy to understand why someone would embrace the idea that HIV is harmless, or that their positive HIV test means nothing, or that they can remain healthy without taking medications. People who are facing a debilitating and life threatening illness are not always in the best state-of-mind to be critical thinkers, ask questions about where their information came from and how it is known to be credible. Sometimes simply reflecting back what a person is saying can help them hear how nutty it sounds. And even when someone goes down the road of denialism, it is important that they are not shunned or abandoned.

The rude awakening of illness dealt by HIV infection does invariably come to those people it afflicts, often snapping them back to realty and out of denialism. Perhaps the best we can do is simply to be there for them when they come back to realism. Talking about AIDS and the real challenges it brings is the one thing that we can all do to bring about the day when we can say "those guys are no longer still around."

Epilogue
The Most Ironic Conspiracy

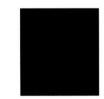

"Once again I would like to suggest that you inform yourself as extensively as possible about the AIDS epidemic. Again, for this purpose, I would recommend that you access the Internet."

Former President Thabo Mbeki, South Africa

On September 22, 2008, with a tally of 2.6 million and counting South Africans having died from AIDS, Thabo Mbeki resigned from the Presidency of South Africa. I just happened to be in Cape Town. After a stunning turn of political events, it seemed that perhaps now South Africa's government may no longer be bogged down by AIDS denialism and perhaps it would accelerate access to the HIV treatments that this country so desperately needs. South Africans had no reason to believe that President Mbeki would ever renounce AIDS denialism and his legacy of slow action on AIDS would surely endure. In response to the President's resignation, AIDS activist Zackie Achmat stated that Mbeki's "culpability in the death of hundreds of thousands of people in South Africa with HIV/AIDS cannot be underestimated and its impact will be felt for generations".

The day after President Mbeki resigned from office, several of his government ministers followed in mass exodus. But not Health Minister Manto Tshabalala-Msimang who had been responsible for instituting South Africa's denialist AIDS policies under Mbeki. It seemed that nothing about South Africa's AIDS crisis would improve soon. Yet later in the same week the newly appointed President Kgalema Motlanthe, in one of his first acts on his first day as President of South Africa, removed the Health Minister from her post. As the new Minister of Health, President Motlanthe named a progressive thinking AIDS realist named Barbara Hogan. The new Minister of Health was literally serenaded at her doorstep by AIDS activists. If you ever wondered how it would feel to be in a place where an oppressive regime was removed from power, this must have been it – at least for those South Africans who care about AIDS. The front pages of Cape Town's newspapers headlined: *"Joy as Manto Leaves Post"*, *"AIDS Activists Serenade New Health Minister as Tshabalala-Msimang Changes Jobs"* and *"Manto Axed from Health"*. Cape Town's evening paper, The Cape Argus informed us that "not a favourable word about the former Health Minister was uttered by MPs [members of parliament]" as she departed.

The man who at this moment seems most likely to be South Africa's next president, former Deputy President Jacob Zuma, had been the Chairperson of the South African National AIDS Council from 1999 to 2005, the years that denialism hijacked South African AIDS policies. As discussed in Chapter 5, Jacob Zuma had also been charged and acquitted of sexually assaulting an HIV positive woman in 2005. During his trial he famously stated that he did not use a condom but rather showered after sex "so it would minimize the risk of contracting the disease". It should not surprise us if President Mbeki and his Health Ministers departures do not lead to rapid reform of South Africa's AIDS policies. It's not like US AIDS policies suddenly became progressive when President Reagan's second term ended. It is foolish indeed to think that AIDS denialism is attributable to any single person.

The ramifications of AIDS denialism felt in South Africa are growing in America as well. Angela Hutchinson and her colleagues at the Centers for Disease Control reported research that showed nearly half of all gay men surveyed in four US cities agreed with the statement "HIV does not cause AIDS". These astounding research findings show that AIDS denialism continues to undermine efforts to test and treat people who are at greatest risk for HIV/AIDS. And it is not just AIDS prevention and treatment that denialism corrupts. Denialism is born from desperation and shows its deceptive face to all life-threatening diseases. The similarities in all forms of medical denialism are actually quite striking, particularly their reliance on pseudoscience and the Internet. We even see the same characters crossing over the fringes of one disease to another disease. Peter Duesberg and David Rasnick, for instance, have turned their attention away from AIDS toward cancer, proclaiming that cancer has no genetic basis just as AIDS has nothing to do with a virus. David Crowe, President of the Rethinking AIDS Society, directs much of his attention to cancer where he promotes 'non-toxic' alternatives to chemotherapies. He says that chemotherapies are deadlier than cancer, exactly what he says about AZT and AIDS. David Crowe also states that cancer treatments are pushed by a conspiracy of medicine, government and Big Pharma, just as AIDS treatments are. He warns us about the conspiracy behind early cancer detection, suggesting that early detection is motivated by financial interests of the cancer industry. He even advocates for the elimination of the profitable profession of oncology – the cancer specialty in medicine. Really? Eliminate oncology? With what alternative? Would he suggest consulting a freelance journalist if you detect a lump in your neck? If AIDS denialism can be held responsible for hundreds of thousands of deaths, as suggested by activist Zackie Achmat, then there is no telling how many deaths cancer denialism is causing.

Most of the nutritionists who sell vitamins and snake oil to treat AIDS also sell bogus cancer cures. The US Food and Drug Administration warns us against over 125 fake cures for cancer, and those are just the ones known to cause harm. Pseudoscientific proclamations that shark cartilage can cure cancer because sharks do not get cancer (although sharks actually do get cancer) were disseminated on the Internet and have bled into the mainstream media. The result has been the loss of human lives, not to mention the desecration of entire shark populations. In their 2004 article in the scientific journal *Cancer Research*, Gary Ostrander and his colleagues concluded that;

> successful sale of crude shark cartilage to the public represents a failure of our society to deal with pseudoscience. The stark contrast between the rigor of scientific peer review and the lack of any substantive review in the popular press underscores the failure of our educational and journalistic systems to ingrain the value of intellectual honesty or to promote the ability of the media and public to think critically. The increased power of electronic media has increased the potential harm of pseudoscience, turning what would otherwise be quaint cultural curiosities into potentially serious societal and ecological problems.

And it is not just life-threatening diseases that must contend with medical denialism. In his 2008 book *Autism's False Prophets*, Paul Offit describes pseudoscientists who have claimed that autism is caused by proteins leaking through the intestines (leaky gut) and by the toxic effects of mercury contained in childhood vaccines. The rogue scientist that Paul Offit credits with bringing credibility and media exposure to the theory that vaccines cause Autism is British gastroenterologist Andrew Wakefield. It is fair to say that Andrew Wakefield is to Autism as Peter Duesberg is to AIDS. Parents of autistic children, just like people who test HIV positive and those diagnosed with cancer, are desperate to understand how something so horrible could happen to them. As parents grasp for hope they are persuaded by factual-sounding scams put forth by apparently reputable scientists. And it was not just the parents of Autistic children who are harmed by claims that vaccines cause childhood neurological disorders; vaccine hysteria causes a decline in parents vaccinating their children and resurgences of childhood diseases. Amazingly, we still find more of the same characters who warn against anti-HIV medications and cancer chemotherapy fueling the hysteria against vaccines. Once again David Crowe warns about the hazards of flu vaccines stating in an online magazine article, "In addition to the health risks of mercury (nervous system damage, cognitive and visual effects), allergic reactions or sensitivities may also develop due to other components of the vaccine, including the eggs used to grow vaccines."

Medical hysteria such as that seen in response to vaccines is the mirror image of medical denialism. Denialism stems from desperation whereas hysteria stems from fear. Denialism and hysteria are both psychological defenses that are supposed to make us feel safe. Denialism has us running toward false hopes whereas hysteria has us running away from false threats. AIDS hysteria causes children to be removed from school. Cancer hysteria leads people to stop using any number of household cleaners and food additives depending on the news story of the day. Breast implant hysteria caused women to dangerously remove perfectly safe prosthetics from their bodies. Vaccine hysteria resulted in a backsliding of immunization programs. For both denialism and hysteria, the appeal to people facing a devastating medical condition is obvious and the opportunities for exploitation are endless.

In describing the events that led to Autism denialism and vaccine hysteria, Paul Offit reflects back on breast implant hysteria, telling us that the "alliance among fringe scientists, personal-injury lawyers, and advocacy groups; the promotion of bad science; the cottage industry of unnecessary tests and lucrative consulting fees, and the accusation that scientists who publicly had exonerated breast implants were part of a massive conspiracy funded by industry. . ." was only to be repeated in response to theories that mercury in vaccines causes autism. And the same can be said about AIDS denialism and cancer denialism. All medical denialism can be summed up as pseudoscientists, freelance journalists, lawyers, and cottage industries all pointing to medical–government–industry conspiracies. Thus, could it be that AIDS denialism, cancer denialism, autism denialism, and the other forms of medical denialism are all part of one movement to promote public distrust in science and medicine? All denialists say diseases are caused by man's own doing, by vaccines, chemicals, drugs, and poverty – not by nature's intelligent design. Denialists offer natural remedies, anti-oxidants and vitamins as cures. They publish their pseudoscientific findings in the very same sham medical journal. All denialists play victim of censorship inflicted by the scientific establishment. They propagate their strange ideas on the unfiltered Internet. They hire lawyers to litigate civil cases against physicians, mainstream scientists, and pharmaceutical companies. With all denialists having so much in common, could this be the greatest irony of all; conspiracy theorizing denialists conspiring against science and medicine? Now that would be something worth blogging about.

Appendix A
Timeline of HIV/AIDS Denialism

Year	US AIDS Cases	Milestone in AIDS	Milestone in Denialism
1981	88	CDC reports first cases of AIDS in New York and California	Australian Perth Group claims that it was established, formulating a theory that AIDS is caused by oxidation
1982	450	California – first baby diagnosed with AIDS linked to blood transfusion	HEAL is established in New York as a supportive agency to people with AIDS.
1984	7,700	Robert Gallo and Luc Montagnier discover the AIDS virus The Gallo/Heckler press conference is held	Casper Schmidt writes first dissenting view on AIDS in the *Journal of Psychohistory* "The Group Fantasy Origins of AIDS"
1985	16,000	AIDS is formally defined in Africa Rock Hudson dies of AIDS	President Ronald Reagan mentions AIDS for the first time in a press conference Freelance journalist John Lauristen publishes series of articles in New York Native critical of HIV research
1986	29,000	First World AIDS Day	President Ronald Reagan urges public not to panic
1987–1988	50,000	AZT is approved by the FDA to treat HIV infection	Duesberg publishes major scientific paper that questions the role of HIV

(continued)

(continued)

Year	US AIDS Cases	Milestone in AIDS	Milestone in Denialism
		National Academy of Sciences determines evidence is sufficient to definitely conclude HIV causes AIDS President Reagan delivers first speech on AIDS *Science* publishes Blattner, Gallo et al.'s article HIV causes AIDS	in causing AIDS in *Cancer Research* *Science* publishes Duesberg's article "HIV is not the cause of AIDS."
1990–1991	206,000	Ryan White dies of AIDS Magic Johnson announces he is HIV positive Freddy Mercury of the rock band Queen dies of AIDS	Former President Ronald Reagan apologizes for neglecting AIDS John Lauristen publishes book *Poison by Prescription: AZT* Robert Root-Bernstein questions whether enough evidence exists to conclude that HIV causes AIDS The Group for the Scientific Reappraisal of the HIV-AIDS Hypothesis is founded
1993	360,000	CDC expands the definition of AIDS to include severe immune suppression – accounting for large jump in AIDS cases	The Perth Group publishes an article in *Biotechnology* that questions the validity of HIV tests due to the "lack of a gold standard"
1995–1996	580,000	FDA approves protease inhibitor drug to treat HIV Announcement that three drug combination therapy effectively slows HIV and improves health FDA approves tests for measuring HIV viral load	Alive and Well AIDS Alternatives is formed by Christine Maggiore Group for the "Scientific Reappraisal of the HIV/AIDS Hypothesis" publishes letter in *Science* stating "We propose that a thorough reappraisal of the

Year	US AIDS Cases	Milestone in AIDS	Milestone in Denialism
		Time magazine names AIDS scientist David Ho Man of the Year	existing evidence for and against this hypothesis be conducted by a suitable independent group. We further propose that critical epidemiological studies be devised and undertaken"
		Research is published showing that AZT dramatically reduces the transmission of HIV from pregnant women to newborns	
		NIH holds consensus conference on HIV prevention and concludes science-based HIV prevention is effective	Duesberg publishes his manifesto, *Inventing the AIDS Virus* with a forward by Kary Mullis, Nobel Prize winner in Chemistry
1998–1999	690,000	Treatment Action Campaign is formed in South Africa to fight for HIV treatment access	Alberta Reappraising AIDS Society is founded and serves as a denialist clearinghouse on the Internet
		President Bill Clinton announces commitment to find an HIV vaccine within 10 years	ACTUP San Francisco is formed as a vocal denialist activist group
2000	775,000	Durban Declaration is published in *Nature*	South African Presidential AIDS Advisory Panel is formed which includes half HIV/AIDS denialists
		International AIDS conference held in Durban South Africa	South African President Mbeki expresses doubt that HIV causes AIDS at International AIDS Conference
			Rebuttal to Durban Declaration published in *Nature*
2001	816,000	President Bush Announces emergency plan for AIDS relief, treating millions for HIV/AIDS	Prominent AIDS denialist group ACTUP San Francisco's David Pasquarelli dies at age 36

(continued)

(continued)

Year	US AIDS Cases	Milestone in AIDS	Milestone in Denialism
		South African AIDS activist Nkosi Johnson dies at age 12	
2004–2005	980,000	New classes of HIV treatments can impact the virus at multiple stages of its life-cycle, including entering a cell 25 years since first reported AIDS cases	Vice President Cheney is asked about the AIDS epidemic among African American women and replies "I have not heard those numbers with respect to African-American women. I was not aware that it was – that they're in epidemic" The biography of Peter Duesberg *"Oncogenes, Aneuploidy, and AIDS: A Scientific Life and Times of Peter H. Duesberg"* is published by Harvey Bialy Christine Maggiore's 3-year-old daughter, Eliza Jane Scovill, dies
2006–2008	Over 1 Million US AIDS Cases and over 30 million in the world	Male circumcision is shown to prevent HIV transmission Bono's Product (Red) campaign raises $47 Million to fund HIV treatment in Africa Leading scientists publish an extensive fact check on Farber's Harper's magazine article, citing more than 50 serious errors FDA approves new class of HIV treatments – Integrase Inhibitors French researchers Francoise Barre-Sinoussi	Gambian President Yahya Jammeh announces he has discovered a cure for AIDS. The herbal treatment was revealed to him by his ancestors in a dream *Harper's* magazine publishes Celia Farber's HIV/AIDS denialist story "Out of Control" Henry Bauer publishes his book, *Origins, Persistence, and Failings of the HIV/AIDS Theory* President Thabo Mbeki of South Africa fires his progressive Deputy

Year	US AIDS Cases	Milestone in AIDS	Milestone in Denialism
		and Luc Montagnier win Nobel Prize for discovering HIV South African President Thabo Mbeki is forced to resign	Minister of Health Nozizwe Madlala-Routledge and this same year discusses his continued HIV/AIDS "dissidence" since 1999 South African courts find Matthias Rath's vitamin studies unlawful *Discover Magazine* publishes full feature article on Peter Duesberg

Appendix B
About the HIV/AIDS Denialists

The major figures in HIV/AIDS denialism are those characters who widely disseminate "dissident" information on AIDS, often creating or fueling conspiracy theories, AIDS myths, and disinformation. To accrue a list of the most notorious HIV/AIDS denialists, I polled a group of AIDS scientists and activists involved with the anti-denialist website www.AIDSTruth.org. I also asked prominent HIV/AIDS denialists for their opinions on who are the most central people among the "HIV=AIDS dissidents." Remarkably, there was a great deal of agreement between the two lists, primarily because the universe of vocal and visible HIV/AIDS denialists is quite small. There was a sentiment among the denialists that those who had risked their career or somehow placed themselves in jeopardy in the name of truth and science were worthy of being prominent in the world of HIV/AIDS denialism.

HIV/AIDS Denialist Scientists

Peter H. Duesberg is the single most important figure in HIV/AIDS denialism because he is the only credentialed scientist who has worked with retroviruses, although not having worked with HIV, to propose that HIV does not cause AIDS. In every respect, HIV/AIDS denialism starts and ends with Peter Duesberg. He is a Professor of Molecular and Cell Biology at the UC Berkeley. He received his PhD in chemistry from the University of Frankfurt in 1963. He is the son of two medical doctors; his father was a professor of internal medicine and doctor in the German army during World War II – something in which he apparently takes no pride. He joined the faculty at Berkley in 1964 and isolated the first cancer gene through his work on retroviruses in 1970. His subsequent work on cancer genes or oncogenes resulted in his election to the prestigious National Academy of Sciences in 1986. However, Duesberg abandoned his research on oncogenes and became a proponent of a cancer theory based on Aneuploidy, an abnormal number of chromosomes. Duesberg claims, counter to mainstream cancer research, that Aneuploidy is the sole cause of cancer. According to Duesberg, chemicals found in food and drugs cause Aneuploidy. In direct parallel, Duesberg challenges that consumption of recreational drugs and medications prescribed to treat HIV are the cause of AIDS. There is great similarity between Duesberg's view that the environment causes cancer without genetic involvement and his theory that toxic drugs and poverty cause AIDS. Both ideas counter established science and are cozy to intelligent design, the new creationism; man is responsible for these terrible ills, which do not reflect defects in God's perfect creations. Also like Intelligent Design, Duesberg's ideas refute established science. An early AIDS dissident scientist, Duesberg is the original and driving force in HIV/AIDS denialism because he has not yielded his personal beliefs to the mountains of scientific evidence that HIV causes AIDS. His views on HIV and AIDS logically lead to his more harmful position that antiretroviral therapies are toxic to the immune system and themselves cause AIDS.

Duesberg is experiencing somewhat of a renaissance in his late years. He had his work in cancer featured in 2007 in *Scientific American Magazine* and was featured in a full article spread in the June 2008 issue of *Discover Magazine*, complete with pictures of him in his lab and with his bicycle. Also in 2008, Duesberg received a Clean Hands Award from the Semmelweis Society for being a whistle blower and telling the truth about AIDS.

David Rasnick. According to Celia Farber, David Rasnick is Peter Duesberg's closest collaborator. In public, Rasnick appears to be Duesberg's right hand man. David Rasnick resided in the Bahamas, although he uses a Ft. Lauderdale address, after living in South Africa for more than a year. He has a doctorate degree in chemistry and he has co-authored articles with Duesberg on AIDS. Rasnick has also written articles on Aneuploidy. At one time, he had a visiting scholar appointment with the Department of Molecular and Cell Biology at UC Berkeley (1996–2005), where he worked with Duesberg, although the university retracted his appointment. One thing that Rasnick brings to HIV/AIDS denialism is his background in studying protease – an enzyme that is critical to the process of HIV replication. Although Rasnick has never actually worked with HIV, he has worked with protease – in rats. Rasnick served with Duesberg on the now infamous panel of AIDS experts and denialists convened by South African President Thabo Mbeki in 2000. In fact, Rasnick is credited, or blamed, with convincing Mbeki that there is a need for a scientific debate on the cause of AIDS.

Rasnick's most recent role in AIDS denialism has been as a Senior Researcher with the Rath Foundation of South Africa. He conducted "research" on vitamins as a cure for AIDS. The Rath and Rasnick studies of vitamins for treating AIDS represent one of the darker moments in AIDS pseudoscience.

The South African courts have found the studies unlawful. Unlike Duesberg whose harm to others has come through words, there are accusations that Rasnick crossed the line by doing harm through his pseudoscientific antics with Matthias Rath. He says that he worked with Rath in South Africa to study the effects of vitamins in caring for people with HIV/AIDS. According to Rasnick, the patients were under the care of their usual doctors who merely provided information for research. The Rath Foundation, however, presents the work as an unethical research trial in which people are know to have died. Rasnick is a conspiracy theorist, as nicely illustrated in the following quote,

> The HIV cult has transported AIDS beyond the domain of science and medicine, and into the realm of mythology. The discourse is controlled by powerful individuals and institutions with a professional or financial stake in HIV, who take it upon themselves to be the sole purveyors of 'truth.' Government institutions have compounded the difficulty of arriving at a true understanding of AIDS by doing everything in their power to suppress the views of scientists who disagree with established opinions. . ... President Clinton did his bit to thicken the protective fog encasing the AIDS Blunder. Last summer he declared AIDS to be a risk to the national security of the United States. That action allowed at least three additional federal institutions to play a direct role in maintaining and protecting the fiction of a global AIDS pandemic. These institutions are the Federal Bureau of Investigation (FBI), the Central Intelligence Agency (CIA), and the National Security Agency (NSA). The involvement of the FBI, CIA, and NSA in AIDS represents a far greater threat to our freedoms than to HIV.[1]

Harvey Bialy received his PhD in molecular biology in 1970 from UC Berkeley. In his 36-year career, Harvey Bialy published 27 scientific articles, nearly half of which were editorials in the journal *Nature Biotechnology*, for which he served as one of the junior editors from 1983 to 1996. He was a resident scholar of the Institute of Biotechnology (IBT) of the National Autonomous University of Mexico between 1996 and 2006. At the beginning of 2007, "he was abruptly, with neither prior discussion nor notification, unilaterally and over the protests of several senior scientists at the IBT, 'disassociated' from both of his previous, and long-held positions." Having not conducted any research since the late 1980s, Bialy is known for his biography of Peter Duesberg, titled *Oncogenes, Aneuploidy, and AIDS*. Harvey Bialy has said, "HIV is an ordinary retrovirus. There is nothing about this virus that is unique. Everything that is discovered about HIV has an analogue in other retroviruses that don't cause AIDS. HIV only contains a very small piece of genetic information. There's no way it can do all these elaborate things they say it does."[2]

Kary B. Mullis. I admit that it seems odd to include a Nobel Laureate among the who's who of AIDS pseudoscientists. In 1994, Mullis co-authored the essay "What causes AIDS? It's an open question" and he has appeared in several interviews in which he clearly questions whether HIV causes AIDS. Mullis said, "If there is evidence that HIV causes AIDS, there should be scientific documents which either singly or collectively demonstrate that fact, at least with a high probability. There is no such document."[3]

Mullis is widely held as an eccentric who has shared his experiences, including his abduction by extraterrestrials. One account of Mullis' erratic behavior comes from John F. Martin who was President of the European Society for Clinical Investigation in the early 1990s:

> Dr. Kary Mullis, who won the Nobel Prize for chemistry in 1993, was invited to speak at the 28th Annual Scientific Meeting of the European Society for Clinical Investigation in Toledo during April. Just before the lecture, he told me he would not speak about the PCR but would tell his ideas about AIDS not being caused by the HIV virus. His talk was in style rambling and in content inappropriate for a public appearance of a leader of science, especially with several hundred young scientists present. His only slides (on what he called "his art") were photographs he had taken of naked women with colored lights projected upon their bodies. He accused science of being universally corrupt with widespread falsification of data to obtain grants. Finally, he impugned the personal honesty of several named scientists working in the HIV field. His own explanation for the immunodeficiency syndrome was incoherent and insubstantial. As chairman, I stopped the lecture after half an hour and asked him to answer three specific questions about the transmission of AIDS to hemophiliacs and from mother to child. His reply was again inappropriate both intellectually and in style. Mullis several times insisted that having won the Nobel Prize gave him authority to speak. Surely, the credible authority of a Nobel laureate should be confined to the subject for which he won the prize (in Mullis's case, chemistry). Mullis not only decreased the nobility of the prize but his attitude was, I believe, a potential corrupting influence on young scientists: among other things, for example, he claimed himself to have changed data-points so as to make data-sets appear more significant by way of illustrating that the practice is a common one.[4]

Charles Geshekter is emeritus professor of African history at California State University, Chico. He was one of the original signatories to the letter that established the Group for the Scientific Reappraisal of the HIV/AIDS Hypothesis. From 2000 to 2003, he was a member of the South African Presidential AIDS Advisory Panel. Geshekter appears to be among the more influential contributors to South African President Mbeki's own ideas on AIDS. Apparently, Geshekter's influence on Mbeki came from his connecting AIDS to racism and colonialism, as illustrated by the following statement:

> The real threats to African lives are famine, rural poverty, migratory labor systems, urban crowding, the collapse of state structures and the sadistic violence of civil wars. When essential services for water, power or transport break down, public

sanitation deteriorates and tuberculosis, dysentery and respiratory infections increase... The best predictors for 'AIDS' anywhere in Africa are economic deprivation, malnutrition, poor sanitation and parasitic infections, not extraordinary sexual behavior or antibodies for a virus that has proved difficult to isolate directly. Journalists should familiarize themselves with the contradictions, anomalies and inconsistencies in the biomedical dogma about HIV/AIDS. Once they consider the non-contagious explanations for 'AIDS' cases in Africa, they can stop the relentless proliferation of terrifying misinformation that equates sexuality with death.[5]

Claus Koehnlein. A German physician, Koehnlein affiliated with the Department of Oncology at the University of Kiel until 1993. Also on the 2000 South African Presidential AIDS Panel, he has only one scientific publication to his credit and it is co-authored with Peter Duesberg and David Rasnick. Koehnlein has mostly directed attention to the harms of HIV medications. According to journalist Celia Farber, Koehnlein has testified as an expert witness in legal cases defending parents who refuse to treat their HIV infected children with antiretroviral (ARV) medications. Koehnlein has, however, been more of a liability than an asset to HIV/AIDS denialism. His statement that people treated with ARVs remain healthy is inconsistent with Peter Duesberg's claim that the medications are toxic. In addition, Koehnlein has said that one of Duesberg's central premises, that ARV medications cause AIDS, can be easily empirically tested and yet is obviously false because there are tragic numbers of children who have never taken illicit drugs and never treated with AZT who have died of AIDS:

> Intoxication hypotheses are easily testable and in contrast to the virus or prion hypotheses also falsifiable. They can be examined toxicologically and epidemiologically and then we can either accept or reject them. For AIDS, the intoxication hypothesis would make following predictions: All patients who die young of AIDS, must have used recreational or antiviral drugs over a longer period. There must not be a significant number of people who die of AIDS at a young age and who are drug free and haven't taken any antivirals.[6]

The Perth Group. When Duesberg was just formulating his dissident views on cancer and AIDS, a small group of Australians was already claiming that HIV does not exist at all. Eleni Papadopulos-Eleopulos, a medical physicist based at the Royal Perth Hospital published a paper in 1988 declaring that HIV had never been correctly isolated as a distinct "pure" virus. The Perth Group also includes Valendar Turner and John Papadimitriou, and they define themselves by taking the following 10 positions in opposition to established AIDS science: failure to prove the existence of a unique, exogenously acquired retrovirus, HIV; failure to verify that HIV antibody tests prove HIV infection; failure to prove HIV causes immune deficiency (destruction of T4 lymphocytes) or AIDS; the impossibility of hemophiliacs acquiring HIV following factor VIII infusions; failure to prove the HIV genome (RNA or DNA) originates in a unique exogenously acquired infectious retroviral particle; failure to prove HIV/AIDS is infectious, either by blood, blood products or sexual intercourse; failure to prove that HIV causes AIDS in Africa or Thailand or is sexually transmitted; that AIDS and all the phenomena inferred as "HIV" are induced by changes in cellular redox brought about by the oxidative nature of substances and exposures common to all the AIDS risk groups and to the cells used in the "culture" and "isolation" of HIV; that AIDS will not spread outside the original risk groups and that cessation of exposure to oxidants and/or use of anti-oxidants will improve the outcome of AIDS patients; and that pharmacological data prove AZT cannot kill HIV and AZT is toxic to all cells and may cause AIDS.

Like Peter Duesberg, the Perth Group claims that drugs, poverty, and HIV medications cause AIDS. They also broaden their view by claiming other sources of immune suppression can lead to AIDS, such as repeated exposure to semen among gay men, although seemingly not women. The Perth Group proposes that an oxidation process occurs in response to HIV/AIDS risk factors, such as drug use, malnutrition, and exposure to semen that causes immune suppression and ultimately AIDS. Although oxidation such as those described by the Perth Group can have important impact for the immune system, there is no evidence that any such processes cause AIDS.

Remarkably, Papadopulos-Eleopulos testified at an appeals hearing for a man who was fighting a conviction for sexually infecting women with HIV who were unaware of his HIV status. In 2007, more than 20 years since she first refuted AIDS science, Papadopulos-Eleopulos testified that HIV is harmless, claiming there were no grounds for charging the defendant. Papadopulos-Eleopulos testified but the Australian court later found her not qualified to express opinions about the existence of HIV.

Etienne de Harven retired from the University of Toronto and having been a Professor of Cell Biology at Sloan Kettering Institute, New York from 1956 to 1981. de Harven isolated and conducted electron microscopic studies of the murine (mouse) friend leukemia virus. He was also a member of the 2000 South Africa's Presidential AIDS Advisory Panel and is a recognized leader among AIDS Rethinkers. He worked as a scientist in his field from the 1950s until he retired. He challenged the proof that HIV has been isolated, according to the standards laid down by him. de Harven has said, "Dominated by the media, by special pressure groups and by the interests of several pharmaceutical companies, the AIDS establishment efforts to control the disease lost contact with open-minded, peer-reviewed medical science since the unproven HIV/AIDS hypothesis received 100% of the research funds while all other hypotheses were ignored."[7]

Roberto Giraldo has a medical degree from the University of Antioguia in Columbia, South America. He was a medical technologist in New York before returning to South America. Roberto Giraldo is most infamous for having conducted a bogus "experiment" where he intentionally incorrectly performed HIV antibody tests to yield false positive results. He claims that HIV may not even exist, and if it does exist, HIV does not cause AIDS. Based on his own pseudoscience, Giraldo has said,

> HIV tests are meaningless. A person can react positive even though he or she is not infected with HIV. The tests are interpreted differently in different countries, which means that a person who is positive in Africa (or Thailand) can be negative when tested in Australia. There is no justification for the fact that most people have not been informed about the serious inaccuracy of the tests. The error has catastrophic repercussions on thousands of people. Since people are reacting positive on tests that are not specific for HIV, let's please stop labeling them as HIV positive.[8]

Mohammed Al-Bayati received his Bachelors of Science from the University of Baghdad, College of Veterinary Medicine in 1975. His training then took him to the University of Cairo where he completed his Masters Thesis titled "Histopathological and histochemical changes in the adrenal glands of the Egyptian Buffalo with follicular cysts and inactive ovaries." Al-Bayati jumped species from non-humans to humans, and he received his doctorate from the UC Davis in Human Pathology, Toxicology, Immunology, and Biochmestry. In addition to being an expert consultant on adverse reactions to vaccines, including anthrax vaccines, Al-Bayati is an AIDS pseudoscientist. The limited research he has published has been nearly exclusively on rats and mice. He has never conducted research on HIV or on humans. Still, he claims that HIV is harmless and that everything from crack cocaine, alkyl nitrites, malnutrition, AZT, and protease inhibitors cause AIDS. Al-Bayati is most notorious for his critique of the Los Angeles County coroner's report for Eliza Jane Scovill, Christine Maggiore's three-year-old daughter who died of AIDS. In one of the more obscene Internet postings in HIV/AIDS denialism, Al-Bayati has exploited the deaths of children by printing their autopsy reports in a dubious journal and posting the reports online.[9]

Lynn Margulis is Distinguished Professor in the Department of Geosciences, University of Massachusetts – Amherst and elected to the National Academy of Sciences in 1983. In 1999, President Clinton presented her with the National Medal of Science, America's highest honor for scientific achievement, "for her outstanding contributions to understanding of the development, structure, and evolution of living things, for inspiring new research in the biological, climatological, geological and planetary sciences, and for her extraordinary abilities as a teacher and communicator of science to the public." Margulis is an accomplished scientist whose endorsement of

HIV/AIDS denialism defies understanding. Margulis has concluded, "I'm not convinced that the various AIDS tests are proof of infection by HIV because I cannot find any study that documents HIV being purified. Given the manufacturers' disclaimers on these products, their use as diagnostic tools is clearly off label. I wonder if this fact is shared with people being given their status as HIV+." Most recently, Professor Margulis has revealed that she is also a 9/11 Truth Seeker, expressing concern that the 9/11 attacks were orchestrated by the Bush Administration to justify the wars in Afghanistan and Iraq, saying, "the 9/11 tragedy is the most successful and most perverse publicity stunt in the history of public relations".[10]

The late **Serge Lang** is a well-known and well-respected mathematician. He was on the faculty of Yale University and became a vocal activist for academic freedom. He also spent time at UC Berkeley and came to know Duesberg. Lang descended into HIV/AIDS denialism and protested what he saw as the unjust treatment of Duesberg. He conducted a flawed analysis of Duesberg's grant failings and called into question the entire NIH review process. He also caused a bit of commotion on the Yale campus when AIDS speakers visited. He protested the appointment of former Global AIDS Program Director at the World Health Organization Michael Merson as Yale's Dean of Public Health and launched a series of letter writing campaigns to Yale administrators about the role the university was playing the global AIDS conspiracy.

Rebecca Culshaw is former a mathematics teacher at the University of Texas Tyler who obtained her doctorate from Dalhousie University in 2002. In graduate school, Culshaw worked with a well-respected researcher, Shigui Ruan on developing mathematical models of the immunological aspects of HIV infection. I want to emphasize that Ruan does not himself deny that HIV causes AIDS. In fact, Ruan has had little contact with his former student since she graduated and cannot be held responsible for her divergence into denialism. In 2006, Culshaw became dissatisfied with the evidence for HIV causing AIDS and abandoned the work she had started in graduate school. She first announced her rethinking AIDS in an essay published on the Lew Rockwell Internet site titled "Why I quit HIV" which she then turned into her book *Science Sold Out: Does HIV Really Cause AIDS?* in which she summarized the denialist positions of the 1980s. Culshaw received the Superior AIDS Rethinking Action Honours from the Alberta Reappraising AIDS Society, although she does not list this achievement on her curriculum vitae.[11]

Henry H. Bauer is Professor Emeritus of Chemistry and Science Studies and Dean Emeritus of Arts and Sciences at the Virginia Polytechnic Institute and State University. Born in Austria, he has held academic positions at the Universities of Sydney, Michigan, Southampton, and Kentucky. He has taught in humanities, science and technology but has never done any notable research of his own. As one of his colleagues told me, Bauer does not have any scientific accomplishments, but he was an able administrator and dean. He has been Editor-in-Chief of the *Journal of Scientific Exploration,* which publishes pseudoscience on everything from alien abductions to telepathy. Before setting out to prove that HIV does not cause AIDS, he was a leading authority on the existence of the Loch Ness Monster. Bauer also has a history of homophobia from which he now claims to be recovering. In 2007, Bauer published *The Origin, Persistence, and Failings of HIV/AIDS Theory,* detailing his wacky methods for determining that HIV does not cause AIDS.[12]

HIV/AIDS Denialist Activists and Journalists

Christine Maggiore is founder of Alive & Well, perhaps the most visible and visited HIV/AIDS denialist website. I have seen several versions of her story, but what seems clear is that she tested for HIV repeatedly with conflicting results. She claims to be HIV positive, untreated, and perfectly healthy. She is therefore most likely one of many long term slow progressors living with HIV. Adding to the confusion, her 3-year-old daughter Eliza Jane Scovill died of complications of AIDS whereas second opinions state that the death was the result of an adverse reaction to antibiotics. Maggiore founded Alive & Well in 1995 and wrote *What If Everything You Thought You Knew about AIDS Was Wrong?* She is married to Robin Scovill, who directed the HIV/AIDS denialist documentary *The Other Side of AIDS,* produced by Robert Leppo who has also financially backed Peter Duesberg's Aneuploidy research lab and conferences.

Celia Farber is a journalist who has chronicled the Peter Duesberg phenomenon since the late 1980s. She was a girlfriend of Bob Guccione, the founder of *Penthouse Magazine* and owner of Penthouse Media Group, Inc. affording Farber considerable access to the publishing world. In 1987, Farber began writing and editing a monthly investigative feature column "Words from the Front" in *SPIN Magazine,* owned by Guccione. She has been featured in *Discover Magazine,* also owned by Guccione. These articles focused on the critiques of HIV/AIDS science. In 2006, she published an article "Out of control: AIDS and the corruption of medical science" in *Harper's* magazine which stirred interest as the article represented a breakthrough of HIV/AIDS denialism into mainstream media. The article is also a chapter in her book, *Serious Adverse Events: An Uncensored History of AIDS,* a collection of her magazine articles, mostly from the 1980s and 1990s. Farber has taken Duesberg on as a cause and in so doing has engaged in several rather nasty exchanges with AIDS scientists, most notably Robert Gallo. Along with Duesberg, Farber received a 2008 Clean Hands Award from the Semmelweis Society for her speaking out about the truth in AIDS.

John Lauritsen is among the earliest critics of how CDC reported HIV/AIDS statistics. He refutes sexual transmission of HIV and believes that drugs cause AIDS. As a gay HIV/AIDS denialist, some gay communities criticize him while others support him. Lauristen once said,

> The crimes against humanity committed in the AIDS War rank with any in history. It takes a while for the enormity of the situation to sink in: that at this very moment, a quarter of a million people are being murdered by nucleoside analogue therapy. ... There are those in the AIDS establishment who know exactly what they are doing, and are profiting thereby. If there were justice in the world, the AIDS-criminals would be brought to justice, given fair trials, and executed. The important thing now is to get out the truth. We must save lives, stop the squandering of our national resources, and rescue the good name of science.[13]

Tom Bethell is a conservative journalist and a senior editor of *The American Spectator* magazine. He writes on a broad range of topics, although he has a particular interest in intelligent design (the new creationism), global warming denial and HIV/AIDS denialism. Unlike most HIV/AIDS denialists, Bethell has a large audience in his following of conservative religious groups. In addition to gravitating to alternative views on AIDS, Bethell is also a proponent of Duesberg's Aneuploidy theory of cancer. In an *American Spectator* magazine article in 2000, Bethell blended conservative rhetoric on AIDS with AIDS pseudoscience, citing some of the more inaccurate misuses of AIDS science, such as

> A sub-Saharan male-and-female AIDS epidemic implies that Africans have abandoned themselves to reckless sexual promiscuity. Recreational drug use is not alleged, and it is well established that it takes a thousand sexual contacts on average to transmit HIV heterosexually. That is why HIV has stayed confined to risk groups in the West. Fables of insatiable African truck-drivers and rampant prostitution – Beverly Hills morals imputed to African villagers – are attempts to rationalize the equal-gender epidemiology of AIDS in Africa. Moslem countries to the north are less likely to accept this libel, so we may predict that the "epidemic" will remain firmly sub-Saharan. Cairo is a river's journey away from the Uganda hotbeds, and yet WHO reports a demure cumulative total of 215 cases in Egypt (pop. 65 million) since AIDS began.[14]

David Crowe is a Canadian journalist based in Alberta and is the founder of the Alberta Reappraising AIDS Society and the President of the Rethinking AIDS Society. He manages the most visible and up-to-date AIDS pseudoscience website on the Internet, which posts numerous clippings from scientific journals out of original contexts and in support of denialist claims. He has long been involved in environmental-naturalist movements and is the founder of the Green Party of Alberta. He is also a prominent agent of disinformation about cancer chemotherapy. Crowe is on the advisory council of Another Look, an organization designed to distribute disinformation on HIV transmission through breastfeeding. Crowe is a signing author on numerous letters and documents refuting HIV/AIDS science. He himself is not, however, a scientist and describes himself as a telecommunications consultant, environmentalist, critic of science and medicine. The aim of his efforts is to free science from the corrupting influence of money.

Notes

1 HIV/AIDS Denialism Is Alive and Well

1. As a life-threatening disease, cancer involves denial as an initial step in coping. The National Cancer Institute (NCI) offers a detailed description of denial available at the NCI web site: http://www.cancer.gov/cancertopics/takingtime/page2#A2

2. ibid.

3. Leading psychiatrists and the American Psychiatric Association have been debating the value of an official psychiatric diagnosis for maladaptive denial. The dialogue on this development is available in Letters to the Editor by Pilowski, I. and Spitzer, R. (1993) *American Journal of Psychiatry, 150* (3), 531. See also Walloch, J. et al., (2007). Delusional denial of pregnancy as a special form of Cotard's Syndrome. *Psychopathology, 40,* 61–64.

4. Several people living with HIV/AIDS have listed their stories on a web site called Living without HIV Drugs http://www.livingwithouthiv-drugs.com/. My attempts to contact them were welcomed with considerable openness. I spoke with several of these people, and they had very genuine accounts, regarding their personal decisions to refuse antiretroviral therapies.

5. Robert Root Bernstein clarified his views on AIDS as evidence grew that HIV does cause immune dysfunction. The statement shown here is from the article "Dead Certain?" by Bob Lederer. Published in POZ magazine April 2006. Accessed at http://en.wikipe dia.org/wiki/Robert_Root-Bernstein

6. Joseph Sonnabend clarified his changing views on AIDS in response to HIV/AIDS denialists continuing to cite his early ideas from the 1980s. The response shown here was retrieved from http://www.aidstruth.org/sonnabend-statement.php, accessed September 29, 2007.

7. A very useful web site on denialism and denialist groups is denialism. com – posted on March 18, 2007. This definition can be found at http:// www.denialism.com/2007/03/what-is-denialism.html. Another useful Internet resource concerning denialism in gene ral is http://www. giveupblog.com/2006/09/denialists.html

8. Liam Sheff posted this statement in a comment for the journal Plos Medicine, available at http://medicine.plosjournals.org/perlserv/?request= read-response&doi=10.1371/journal.pmed.0040256

9. Celia Farber, Out of control: *AIDS and the corruption of medical science. Harper's Magazine, March 2006.*

10. David Rasnick describes his experience at the Gordon Conference on the Chemotherapy of AIDS in March 1997. The story has been recounted on several HIV/AIDS denialist web sites. I quote the account at virusmyth. com, http://www.virusmyth.com/aids/hiv/drconf.htm.

11. Michael Shermer is a leading authority on Holocaust denial. His book *Why People Believe Weird Things: Pseudoscience, Superstition, and Other Confusions of Our Time* published in 2002 by Owl Books is an important source in understanding all denialism. This quote is found on p. 212. The most informative home for Holocaust denialism and the call for a true debate on the history of the Holocaust is located at http://www.ihr.org/ jhr/v01/v01p–5_Butz.html.

12. The Perth Group's statement that they do not deny AIDS is located at the web site http://www.theperthgroup.com/LATEST/response-to-moore.pdf.

13. Stanley Cohen's (2001) book *States of Denial: Knowing About Atrocities and Suffering* provides great insight into the social process of denial. He illustrates how entire societies can enter into denial in response to trauma, such as in the aftermath of war and natural disasters. Mass denial is akin to denial as I have described here and is quite different from denialism.

14. Shapiro, D. (1965). *Neurotic Styles.* Basic Books, p. 56.

15. The AIDS Rethinkers list is posted at www.rethinkingaids.com. The list changes with additions and deletions. It is fairly easy to be included on the list. Requests are made to the webmaster and a follow-up email inquires who you are and why you want to be on the list. A false name is easily included, demonstrating that the authenticity of those on the list is impossible to assess.

16. Shughart, W.F. (2007) Book review "Henry H. Bauer". The Origin, Persistence and Failings of HIV/AIDS Theory. *Public Choice,* Published online.

2 Peter Duesberg and the Origins of HIV/AIDS Denialism

1. Casper Schmidt. (1984). The Group-Fantasy Origins of AIDS *Journal of Psychohistory,* Summer. Accessed at http://www.reviewingaids.com/awiki/index.php/Document:Group-Fantasy_Origins.
2. Peter Duesberg's National Academy of Sciences citation available at http://www.nason line.org/.
3. This quote is from Duesberg, P. (1987). Retroviruses as carcinogens and pathogens: expectations and reality. *Cancer Research,* 47, 1199–1220, page 1202. He made similar comments in other articles; Duesberg, P. (1983). Retroviral transforming genes in normal cells? *Nature,* 304(5923), 219–226. Also, Duesberg, P. (1985). Activated proto-onc genes: sufficient or necessary for cancer? *Science,* 228(4700), 669–677. Duesberg, P. (1989). Human immunodeficiency virus and acquired immunodeficiency syndrome: correlation but not causation. *Proceedings of the National Academy of Science,* 86(3), 755–764.
4. This quote was taken from an interview Peter Duesberg had with the Daily Californian Berkeley campus paper *September 30, 1999* accessed at http://www.dailycal.org/sharticle.php?id=456 retrieved 8/26/07.
5. Editor's note for Peter Duesberg's article in *Scientific American,* "Chromosomal Chaos and Cancer," by Peter Duesberg, May 2007, pp. 52–59.
6. Fox online news article by Steven Milloy, July 8, 2005, "Trillion-Dollar Radiation Mistake?" Accessed at http://www.foxnews.com/story/0,2933,161866,00.html.
7. Gallo quote from Introduction for Peter Duesberg (1984) By Robert C. Gallo *National Cancer Institute, Maryland,* accessed at http://duesberg.com/about/pdintroduction.html.
8. Quote taken from Peter H. Duesberg, 1996, Inventing the AIDS Virus published by Regency, pp. 202–203. Also see Peter Duesberg's book review of Robert Gallo's *Virus Hunting* for the *New York Native* 29 April 1991, retrieved 10/10/07 http://www.virusmyth.net/aids/data/pdhunting.htm.
9. This quote is taken from a talk By Peter H. Duesberg for CAL Alumni on March 6, 1993 accessed at http://www.duesberg.com/about/pdlecture.html.
10. Robert Gallo gave Spin Magazine the first of two interviews with Anthony Liversidge in February 1988 to respond directly to Peter Duesberg's interview with the magazine. This excerpt is taken from

the online printing accessed from the virusmyth.net web site, http://www.virusmyth. com/aids/hiv/alinterviewrg.htm.

11. Randy Shilts *And The Band Played On*, 2000, *Macmillan* p. 367. People who were witness to the early days of AIDS and who knew Randy Shilts have said that the portrayal of good and evil in his book tends to be exaggerated. Nevertheless, this important book is the closest we have to a historical record of the early days of AIDS.

12. Anthony Brink's Debating AZT: The Pope of AIDS. Accessed at http://www.virusmyth. net/aids/data/abpope.htm.

13. Recent research from the Multicenter AIDS Cohort Studies has once again demonstrated that drug use does not cause the immune dysfunction seen in AIDS, where as HIV surely does. See C. Chao, et al. (2008). Recreational drug use and T-lymphocyte subpopulations in HIV-uninfected and HIV-infected men, *Drug and Alcohol Dependence*, *doi: 10.1016/j.drugalcdep.2007.11.010*.

14. From Serge Lang's analysis of Peter Duesberg's NIDA grant review. Lang, S. (1995). To fund or not to fund, that is the question: Proposed experiments on the drug-AIDS hypothesis, to inform or not to inform, that is another question. *Yale Scientific*, Winter. accessed at http://www.virusmyth.net/aids/data/slfund.htm.

15. ibid.

16. Institute of Medicine (1994). AIDS and Behavior: An integrated approach. National Academies Press. The NIH historically funds only a small percentage of grants that are submitted by scientists, typically less than 20% and in many years less than 10%.

17. Awarded grant information available from the NIH http://crisp.cit.nih.gov/crisp/. NIDA grant awarded to E.M Dax, 1Z01DA000014-04 for poppers study. NIDA also awarded a similar grant to Lee Soderberg.

18. Peter Duesberg's whitepaper The African AIDS Epidemic: New and contagious or old under a new name? Addressed to the South African Presidential AIDS Panel, June 22, 2000. Accessed through http://www.duesberg.com/subject/africa2.html.

19. Celia Farber Serious Adverse Events: An uncensored history of AIDS, 2006, Melville House Publishing, p. 49. I should note that it is impossible for Celia Farber or anyone to know who reviews any particular grant. The process is completely protected by rules of confidentiality, as Duesberg himself has complained about. The roster of all the reviews is public, but not the reviewers of a particular grant. For even a couple of biased reviewers to overthrow the entire review process is quite far-fetched. The scenario that Harvey Bialy and Celia Farber portray has the thrill of a good conspiracy theory but is not grounded in reality.

20. David Rasnick, Time to separate state and science, April 2001, accessed at http://www.virusmyth.net/aids/data/drstate.htm 8/14/07.
21. Harvey Bialy, June 2006, The US Government Responds to the 'AIDS Denialist' Writing in the March Harper's by http://www.lewrockwell.com/orig7/bialy5.html.
22. Duesberg, P., Koehnlein, C. ,and Rasnick, D. (2003) The chemical bases of the various AIDS epidemics: recreational drugs, anti-viral chemotherapy and malnutrition, *Journal of Biosciences*, 28(4), 383–412.
23. Peter Duesberg interview with Joseph Mercola, 2001 What If Everything We Thought We Knew about Cancer Was Wrong? Accessed from http://www.reviewingaids.org/awiki/index.php/Document:Mercola_interviews_Duesberg 8/14/2007 also available at http://www.mercola.com/2001/apr/18/duesberg.htm.
24. This quote is taken from the Welcome Address that Peter Duesberg delivered at his second Conference on Aneuploidy and Cancer: Clinical and experimental aspects in Oakland California on February 3, 2008. The exact statement is taken from the opening of the conference program.
25. Cohen, J. (1994). Could drugs, rather than a virus, be the cause of AIDS? *Science, 266*, 1648–1649; Cohen, J. (1994). Duesberg and critics agree: Hemophilia is the best test. *Science, 266*, 1645–1646; Cohen, J. (1994). The Duesberg phenomenon. *Science, 266*, 1642–1644; Cohen, J. (1994). Fulfilling Koch's postulates. *Science, 266*, 1647. These articles are available open access, free at http://www.sciencemag.org/feature/data/cohen/cohen.dtl.
26. O'Brien, S.J. & Goedert, J.J. (1996). HIV causes AIDS: Koch's postulates fulfilled. *Current Opinion in Immunology*, 8, 613–618.
27. See de Lejarazy, R.O., et al. (2008). HIV-1 infection in persistently HIV-1 seronegative individuals: More reasons for HIV RNA screening. *Clinical Infectious Diseases*, 6, 785.

3 AIDS Pseudoscience

1. Editorial, Politics must move mainstream on AIDS. *South African Medical Journal,* March 2003, 93(3).
2. Valendar Turner, What is the evidence for the existence of HIV? Accessed at http://www.virusmyth.net/aids/data/vtevidence.htm.
3. Alexander Russell April 2002 with Perth Group offers a cash reward for isolating HIV. The HUW Christie Memorial Prize $20,000 Reward for 'HIV'. Accessed at http://www.virusmyth.net/aids/news/araward.htm.

4. Roberto Giraldo, June 2000, An effective treatment for AIDS, accessed from http://www.robertogiraldo.com/eng/papers/AnEffectiveTreatment ForAIDS.html accessed 0/17/2007.

5. HIV testing examines whether a person has been exposed to HIV by detecting the presence of antibodies to HIV rather than the presence of the virus itself. Our immune system produces antibodies in response to an invading virus or other agent of disease. Each type of invading particle that the immune system encounters is assigned its own specific antibodies which cannot be confused with antibodies produced for a different invader. This is the lock and key concept that explains why our immune system does not attack our own cells and why we have immunities to diseases we are exposed to more than once. Detecting specific antibodies means that a person has been exposed to a specific disease.

HIV testing involves two stages. First, blood (or saliva) is screened for HIV antibodies using an enzyme-linked immunosorbent assay (ELISA) test. ELISA is one of several techniques available for antibody testing. The ELISA test is done first because it is sensitive to HIV antibodies – if there are HIV antibodies present the ELISA test is likely to detect them. When the ELISA test is negative (i.e., when it does not detect HIV antibodies), it is exceedingly unlikely that the test results are in error, so it is rare for the test to be repeated. However, positive ELISA tests – results that do detect antibodies – are always repeated because in a very small but still important percentage of cases the test can mistakenly pick up non-HIV antibodies. Although rare, false positive ELISA test results do occur. It is for this reason that the ELISA test is used to first screen blood for the presence of HIV antibodies.

Consequently, in the case of a positive ELISA result, it is standard to confirm the HIV positive result with a Western Blot test. Western Blot techniques determine the exact antigens, or parts of HIV, against which the antibodies found in the person, are targeted. A positive Western Blot test result detects HIV antibodies, meaning the identification of two out of three precise HIV antigens. Western Blot specifically tests for the presence of antibodies against three groups of proteins that are part of HIV: (a) the proteins that form the viral envelope, (b) a group of proteins found in the core of the virus, and (c) the polymerase enzyme that is essential for the replication of HIV. To be considered a confirmed HIV positive test result, the Western Blot test must identify at least two of the three antibodies present for a positive Western Blot test. Detection of antibodies against certain viral proteins makes the Western Blot test specific to HIV. It is extraordinarily rare for Western Blot tests to yield a false positive result.

6. Claus Koehnlein, April 27, 2001 BSE/AIDS/Hepatitis C Infectious or Intoxication Diseases? Accessed at the web site http://aidsmyth.addr.com/report/news/010427clauskohnlein.htm.

7. Quote from Rebecca Culshaw, 2007 *Science Sold Out: Does HIV Really Cause AIDS?* p. 25, North Atlantic Publishing in Berkeley CA. Why is invasive cervical cancer included in the expanded AIDS definition? The CDC stated, "Several studies have found an increased prevalence of cervical dysplasia, a precursor lesion for cervical cancer, among HIV-infected women... In addition, HIV infection may adversely affect the clinical course and treatment of cervical dysplasia and cancer." Centers for Disease Control and Prevention, 1993 Revised Classification System for HIV Infection and Expanded Surveillance Case Definition for AIDS Among Adolescents and Adults available at http://www.cdc.gov/MMWR/preview/MMWRhtml/00018871.htm.

8. Neville Hodgkinson, May 21, 2006, The circular reasoning scandal of HIV testing accessed at http://www.thebusinessonline.com.

9. Quote from Bauer, H. H. (2006). Demographic characteristics of HIV: III. Why does HIV discriminate by race? *Journal of Scientific Exploration, 20*(2), 255–288. also available at http://hivnotaids.homestead.com. A more detailed description of AIDS in races is in Henry Bauer's 2007 book *The Origin, Persistence, and Failings of HIV/AIDS Theory*, published by MacFarland.

10. J.W. Bess et al. 1997, Microvesicles are a source of contaminating cellular proteins found in purified HIV-1 preparations. *Virology*, 2, 134–144; P. Gluschankof et al., 1997, Cell membrane vesicles are a major contaminant of gradient-enriched human immunodeficiency virus-1 preparations. *Virology*, 230, 125–133; E. Chertova et al., 2006, Proteomic and biochemical analysis of purified human immunodeficiency virus type 1 produced from infected monocyte-derived macrophages. *Journal of Virology*, 80(18), 9039–9052.

11. R. Culshaw, 2006, Why I Quit HIV accessed at http://www.lewrockwell.com/orig7/culshaw1.html accessed 8/10/07.

12. R. Giraldo, 1999, Everybody Reacts Positive on the ELISA Test for 'HIV'. *Continuum*, 5, 9–11. Continuum was a magazine that served as a dedicated outlet for HIV/AIDS denialism in the late 1990s which as since gone out of business.

13. R. Culshaw, 2007, *Science Sold Out: Does HIV Really Cause AIDS?* p. 25, North Atlantic Publishing in Berkeley, CA.

14. Peter Duesberg interviewed by Joshua Nicholson for *City on a Hill Press*. Article title Is HIV Truly the Cause of AIDS? New Research Could Suggest Otherwise. Accessed at http://www.cityonahillpress.com/article.php?id=631 10/13/2007.

15. Rodriguez response 'What our work means' By Benigno Rodriguez M.D. M.Sc. and Michael M. Lederman M.D. Case Western Reserve University Center for AIDS Research. Accessed at http://www.aidstruth.org/ rodriguez-lederman.php.

16. D. Crowe June 2007, Nice Graph, No Data. Accessed at http://aras.ab.ca/ articles/scientific/DatalessGraphs.html 8/26/2007.

17. H. Bauer referring to his 2007 book *The Origin, Persistence, and Failings of HIV/AIDS Theory*, published by MacFarland on his web site http:// hivnotaids.homestead.com.

18. R. Culshaw, 2007*Science Sold Out: Does HIV Really Cause AIDS?* p. 25, North Atlantic Publishing in Berkeley, CA.

19. Review of The Origin, Persistence, and Failings of HIV/AIDS Theory by Darin Brown http://www.reviewingaids.org/awiki/index.php/Document: Brown_reviews_Bauer 10/14/ 2007.

20. W. F. Shughart 2007, Henry H. Bauer. The Origin, Persistence and Failings of HIV/AIDS Theory. Book Review, *Public Choice*. epub ahead of print, DOI 10.1007/s11127-007-9233-2.

21. H. Bauer's Loch Ness Odyssey, http://www.henryhbauer.homestead. com/ p. 9.

22. T. Bethell, August 17, 1992, COULD DUESBERG BE RIGHT? *National Review*. Accessed at http://www.virusmyth.net/aids/data/tbcould.htm accessed 11/3/2007.

23. P. Dellinger February 28, 2006, Retired professor argues that HIV does not cause AIDS http://www.roanoke.com/news/nrv/wb/wb/xp-54692.

24. Henry Bauer, 2007,*The Origin, Persistence, and Failings of HIV/AIDS Theory*, published by MacFarland, p. 238.

25. Joseph Sonnabend clarified his changing views on AIDS in response to HIV/AIDS denialists continuing to cite his early ideas from the 1980s. The response shown here was retrieved from http://www.aidstruth.org/ sonnabend-statement.php, accessed September 29, 2007.

26. R. Root-Bernstein, 1993, Rethinking AIDS: The Tragic Cost of Premature Consensus, Free Press, Robert Root Bernstein clarified his views on AIDS as evidence grew that HIV does cause immune dysfunction. The statement shown here is from the article "Dead Certain?" by Bob Lederer. Published in POZ magazine April 2006, http://en.wikipedia.org/wiki/ Robert_Root-Bernstein.

27. P. Duesberg, presented at the Lew Rockwell Conference, Foster City, December 1–2, 2006.

28. S. Gregson's study published in the Proceedings of the National Academy of Sciences and summarized in "HIV/AIDS In Zimbabwe Has Reduced Life Expectancy, Not Affecting Population Growth, Study Says" accessed at http://www.medicalnewstoday.com/arti cles/80976.php 10/15/2007.

29. P. Duesberg discussed this study in a presentation and posted slides that included this analysis. The title of the presentation was "A multibillion $ Quiz: Is AIDS a viral or a chemical epidemic?" delivered to the Lew Rockwell Conference in Foster City December 1–2, 2006. The slides were accessed at http://mcb.berkeley.edu/labs/duesberg/.

30. The Antiretroviral Therapy (ART) Cohort Collaboration, 2006, HIV treatment response and prognosis in Europe and North America in the first decade of highly active antiretroviral therapy: a collaborative analysis *Lancet* 2006; 368: 451–58.

31. D. Rasnick, August 2000, Contributions to Mbeki's Expert AIDS Panel Accessed at http://www.virusmyth.net/aids/data/drpanel.htm 8/14/2007.

32. Dr. Rath Health Foundation, 2007, Dark cloud over good works of Gates Foundation. Accessed at http://www4.dr-rath-foundation.org/THE_FOUNDATION/microsoft.htm 10/14/2007.

33. President Thabo Mbeki quoted in Andrew Feinstein, 2007, After the Party: A personal and political journey inside the ANC, Jonathan Ball Publishing, Jeppestown, South Africa.

34. Celia Farber Serious Adverse Events: An uncensored history of AIDS, 2006, Melville House Publishing.

35. J. Bergman (n.d.). Drugs, disease, denial. *New York Press*. Retrieved August 27, 2007, from http://www.nypress.com/18/25/news&columns/berman.cfm; L. Schiff (2005, May 27). Journalism is bad. Message posted to http://liam.gnn.tv/blogs/6445/Journalism_is_bad.

36. A. Brink open letter to Dr Olive Shisana CEO, *Human Sciences Research Council*. Accessed at Treatment Information Group, www.tig.org.za.

37. S. Kruglinski, 2006, Questioning the HIV Hive Mind? An interview with Celia Farber, long-serving chronicler of HIV dissidents. *Discover Magazine*, accessed http://discovermagazine.com/2006/oct/celia-farber-interview-aids/ 2/27/2008.

38. E. Papadopulos-Eleopulos et al., Rethinking AIDS, 2003, HIV in South Africa accessed at http://www.rethinking.org/bmj/response_30348.html 2/27/2008.

39. G. T. Stewart, September 2000, The Durban Declaration is not accepted by all Nature, 407, www.nature.com accessed 2/26/2008.

40. Bauer, H. (2005). Demographic Characteristics of HIV: I. How Did HIV Spread? *Journal of Scientific Exploration*, 19(4), 567–603.

41. Because her work is high profile, important, and funded by the NIH and the Bill and Melinda Gates Foundation, Nancy Padian's research has been misused by nearly every AIDS denialist. Padien's statement http://www.aidstruth.org/nancy-padian.php; Padian NS, Shiboski SC, Glass SO, Vittinghoff E. 1997. Heterosexual transmission of human immunodeficiency virus (HIV) in Northern California: results from a ten-year study. *American Journal of Epidemiology* 146, 350–357.

42. Stuart Brody, 1997, Sex at Risk, Transaction Publishers, pp. 154–155.

43. Quote taken from a reuters news report cited in Edward Hooper, Opposition to the OPV theory (2) The Marx/Drucker theory of iatrogenic spread through unsterile needles, and the recent intervention by Professor David Gisselquist, who claims that most HIV infections in Africa are caused through this same route. Accessed at http://www.uow. edu.au/arts/sts/bmartin/dissent/documents/AIDS/Hooper03/Hooper03 Marx.html. 2/11/08.

44. G. Schmid et al., 2004, Transmission of HIV-1 infection in sub-Saharan Africa and effect of elimination of unsafe injections. *Lancet* 363: 482–88.

45. M.P. Carey and S.C. Kalichman (1995). Heterosexual Transmission of Human Immunodeficiency Virus (HIV) and Condom Efficacy: More Facts than Fictions (Letter). *Archives of Sexual Behavior*, 24, 657–663.

46. Description found at http://www.dr-rath.com/en/products/immunocell. html 10/24/2007.

47. The Wrongs of Matthias Rath and TAC's efforts to stop his harmful activities. http://www.tac.org.za/community/rath accessed 6/9/08.

48. S. Barrett, March 13, 2005, A Critical Look at Gary Null's Activities and Credentials. Accessed at http://www.quackwatch.org/04Consumer Education/null.html accessed 10/18/2007.

4 Denialist Journalism and Conspiracy Theories

1. 9/11 truth web site http://www.crisispapers.org/Editorials/PNAC-Primer.htm.

2. The moon landing hoax web site http://www.apfn.org/apfn/moon.htm.

3. Cristine Maggiore interview on Rethinking AIDS web site http://www. aliveandwell.org/html/rethinking/deconstructing_aids.html.

4. Web vignette from the Body web site http://img.thebody.com/nmai/ 101.pdf.

5. Web vignette from Virus myth web site http://www.virusmyth.net/aids.

6. Culshaw, R. (2007). *Science Sold Out: Does HIV really cause AIDS?* North Atlantic, Berkeley CA. p. 68.

7. Charles Geshekter is quoted in Gary Null's AIDS a Second Opinion, available at http://www.garynull.com/Documents/aids.htm.

8. Answering AIDS denialists and AIDS lies http://www.aidstruth.org/new/ denialism/answering_denialists accessed June 11, 2008.

9. Deconstructing AIDS. Reprinted from an interview for The Sun, April 25, 2004. An Interview with Christine Maggiore By Derrick Jensen http:// www.aliveandwell.org/html/rethinking/deconstructing_aids.html.

10. Anthony Brink writes extensively on HIV/AIDS denialism and anti-HIV treatments. The quoted material and other examples can be accessed at http://www.virusmyth.net/aids/data/abnvp.htm.

11. Technobabble is defined and discussed at the wikipedia web site http://en.wikipedia.org/wiki/Technobabble.

12. Matt Irwin, 2001, False positive viral loads: What Are We Measuring? http://www.virusmyth.net/aids/data/miloads.htm.

13. This widely cited 2000 quote from South African President Mbeki can be found at http://healtoronto.com/mbeki.html.

14. This quote comes from a long rant at the web site http://www.gatago.org/misc/health/aids/52200807.html.

15. Peter Duesberg December 2005, interviewed by David Jay Brown titled Challenging the Viral Theory of AIDS: An Interview with Dr. Peter Duesberg accessed at http://www.smart-publications.com/articles/MOM-duesberg.php.

16. David Crowe, The AIDS Creed, accessed at http://aras.ab.ca/articles/popular/AidsCreed.html.

17. Peter Duesberg quoted in Tom Bethell 17 Aug. 1992 Could Duesberg be Right? National Review. Accessed at http://www.virusmyth.com/aids/hiv/tbcould.htm.

18. Toby Gettins wrote this quote on a BBC new blog titled "Is AIDS killing intimacy?" Available at http://news.bbc.co.uk/2/hi/africa/3257533.stm.

19. Tara Smith and Steven Novella, 2007, HIV Denial in the Internet Era PLoS Med 4(8): e256. Accesed at http://medicine.plosjournals.org/perlserv/?request=get-document
&doi=10.1371%2Fjournal.pmed.0040256.

20. Culshaw, R. (2007). *Science Sold Out: Does HIV really cause AIDS*? North Atlantic, Berkeley CA, p. 49.

21. This quote was widely disseminated. It can be accessed at http://nationalexpositor.com/News/236.html.

22. Detailed account of the Tuskegee Syphilis study is available at the CDC web site http://www.cdc.gov/tuskegee/timeline.htm. Two articles provide excellent accounts of Dr. Wouter Basson ion South Africa, William Finnegan, A Reporter At Large, The Poison Keeper, The New Yorker, January 15, 2001; Niehaus, I. and Jonsson, G. (2001). Dr. Wouter Basson, Americans, and Wild Beasts: Men's conspiracy theories of HIV/AIDS in the South African Lowveld. *Medical Anthropology, 24,* 179–208.

23. Posted by the Dr. Rath Foundation and accessed at http://www.laleva.cc/supplements/rath_042003.html.

24. David Rasnick,June 1997, Blinded by Science, Spin Magazines, accessed at http://www.virusmyth.com/aids/hiv/drblinded.htm.

25. David Crowe maintains the Reappraising AIDS Society web site. Like his views on AIDS, his involvement in cancer is consistent with his anti-establishment frame of reference. This quote and more on Crowe's views on cancer are available at http://www.alive.com/4887a12a2.php?text_page=2 and http://www.alive.com/4887a12a2.php.
26. Paul and Kelly Brennan-Jones, August, 2007, The HIV/AIDS Myth: A Review of Duesberg's Inventing the AIDS Virus. http://www.alaskafree press.com/msgboard/board/613.
27. This quote is taken from the second interview Robert Gallo did with Anthony Liversidge of*Spin Magazine*, March 1989.
28. Taibbi, M. (2008). The great derangement: A terrifying true story of war, politics and religion at the twilight of the American Empire. Spiegel & Grau: New York.
29. Moore, J.P., Bergman, J. and Wainberg, M. (March, 2007). The AIDS Denialists are Still Around. *International AIDS Society Newsletter*, p. 5
30. This quote was taken from an interview with Mark Wainberg that was shown in the HIV/AIDS denialist film*The Other Side of AIDS* that was written and produced and directed by Robin Scovill who is married to Christine Maggiore.

5 Politics of Denialism

1. Margaret Heckler's 2006 interview with PBS Frontline accessed at http://www.pbs.org/wgbh/pages/frontline/aids/interviews/heckler.html accessed 10/10/2007.
2. Peter Duesberg emphasizes the historical significance of the Press Conference in many of his writings and interviews on AIDS. This excerpt is from page 7 of his 1997 book *Inventing the AIDS Virus*, published by Regency.
3. From the Alive and Well web site, A closer look at HIV: Is HIV the Cause of AIDS? Accessed at www.aliveandwell.org/html/a_closer_look/acloserlook.html.
4. Seth Roberts July 1990, LAB RAT, What AIDS Researcher Dr. Robert Gallo Did in Pursuit of the Nobel Prize. Accessed at http://www.virusmyth.net/aids/data/srlabrat.htm.
5. Liam Scheff has a multipart denialist web site at the whale.to web site which is dedicated to the search for the truth (and the fun of exploration) and freedom from Tyranny. This except was accessed at http://www.whale.to/b/scheff_h.html.
6. Culshaw, R. (2007). *Science Sold Out Does HIV really cause AIDS?* North Atlantic books, Berkeley.

7. President Reagan press conference accessed at http://www.aegis.com/topics/timeline/RReagan-091785.html accessed 10/30/2007.

8. President Reagan Congress on America's Agenda for the Future in February 1986. http://www.aegis.com/topics/timeline/RReagan-020686. html. President Reagan American Foundation for AIDS Research (AmFAR) http://www.pbs.org/wgbh/pages/frontline/aids/docs/amfar.html.

9. From the 2004 Vice Presidential debate, broadcast on ABC, accessed at http://www.actupny.org/reports/debateVP2004.html 2/29/2008.

10. Article by Adam Nagourney, McCain Stumbles on HIV Prevention, in The New York Times Politics Blog, March 16, 2007, accessed at http://thecaucus.blogs.nytimes.com/2007/03/16/mccain-stumbles-on-hiv-prevention/ accessed 2/28/2008.

11. See BBC. SA's Zuma 'showered to avoid HIV', April 5, 2006.

12. Dr. Mulberry's statement was printed in the June 26 1997 in the New York Times Magazine and was accessed at http://query.nytimes.com/gst/fullpage.html?res =9B0DEFD71E3DF935A157.

13. Report of the National Institutes of Health Consensus Conference on Interventions to Prevent HIV Risk Behaviors, 1997.

14. President Mbeki's 2000 International AIDS Conference speech accessed at www.info. gov.za/speeches/2000/0005311255p1003.htm. Accessed 10/27/2007.

15. Gevisser, M. (2007). *Thabo Mbeki The Dream Deferred*, Jonathan Ball Publishers, Cape Town. This biography provides an in depth assessment of the man his political career. An entire chapter is dedicated to Mbeki's views on AIDS with details that have never before been revealed.

16. Feinstein, A. (2007). *After the Party: A personal and political journey inside the ANC*. Jonathan Ball Publishers, Jeppestown, South Africa.

17. See http://www.dr-rath.com/en/products/immunocell.html accessed 10/24/2007.

18. There are numerous accounts of the South African Health Minister and her reluctance to provide HIV treatments. One clear account is provided by Clare Kapp in the Lancet, accessed at www.thelancet.com. Vol 366 November 26, 2005. The essential source for denialism in South Africa is Nicoli Nattrass' 2007 book *Mortal Combat: AIDS Denialism and the Struggle for Antiretrovirals in South Africa*, published by KwaZulu Natal University Press.

19. Clare Kapp in the Lancet, accessed at www.thelancet.com. Vol 366. November 26, 2005.

20. See Nattrass, N. (2007). AIDS Denialsim vs. Science. Skeptical Enquirer, September/October, 31–37; Geffen, N. (2006). Echoes of Lysenko: State sponsored pseudo-science in South Africa. *Social Dynamics*, 31, 183–210.

21. Alberta reappraising AIDS Society S.A.R.A.H. – Superior AIDS Rethinking Action Honours accessed at http://www.aras.ab.ca/SARA/sara.html.
22. Nattrass, N. (2004). *The moral economy of AIDS in South Africa.* Cambridge Press, Cambridge.
23. Quoted in Lawson, L. (2008). *Side effects.* Double Storey Publishers. Cape Town, South Africa.
24. The Durban declaration printed in Durban Declaration, *Nature, 2000,* 406, 15–16.
25. President Mbeki's 2000 International AIDS Conference speech accessed at www.info. gov.za/speeches/2000/0005311255p1003.htm 10/27/2007.
26. Stewart, G., et al. (2000). The Durban Declaration is not accepted by all. *Nature,* 407, 286.
27. Silja J.A., February 25, 2000, Foo Fighters, HIV Deniers accessed at http://www. motherjones.com/news/feature/2000/02/foo.html 11/2/2007.
28. This excerpt is from the HEAL web site accessed at http://home.earth-link.net/revdocnyc/
29. The most notable instance of Peter Duesberg referring to gays as homos occur in the June 2008 *Discover* magazine article featuring him and his efforts in cancer.
30. Neville Hodgkinson. May 2006, The Circular Reasoning Scandal of HIV Testing THE BUSINESS. http://www.aidsinfobbs.org/redribbon.htm.
31. Tom Bethell August 17, 1992, Could Duesberg be right? National Review, accesed at http://www.virusmyth.net/aids/data/tbcould.htm 11/3/2007.
32. Bauer, H. (2007). *The Origin, Persistence, and Failings of HIV/AIDS Theory,* MacFarland.
33. Peter Duesberg in Gay Lesbian Times accessed at http://www.gaylesbian-times.com/?id=9919.
34. Delaney, M. (May 2000). HIV, AIDS, and the distortion of science. *FOCUS a Guide to AIDS Research and Counseling.*
35. This excerpt is from Henry Bauer's 1988 book To Rise above Principle *The Memoirs of an Unreconstructed Dean written under the pseudonym* Josef Martin published by University of Illinois Press. The book is out of print and can be accessed at Henry Bauer's web site http://hivnotaids.homestead.com/
36. Anthony Brink excepted from his self-published book *The Trouble with Nevirapine* p. 20.
37. David Crowe sent an email asking for donations to contribute to the defense fund for Andre Parenzee. The email was subject lined AIDS Rethinkers Should Fight to Keep HIV+ People Out of Jail and sent 10/4/07. The except is taken from that email.

6 Getting Out of Denial

1. See Living without HIV drugs web site http://www.livingwithouthiv-drugs.com/
2. Excerpts from posting in response to the story "AIDS Denialists Disinvited From Congressional Hearing – but Get Indirect Endorsement From Rep. Sheila Jackson Lee" at http://www.thebody.com/content/whatis/art46788.html, accessed 6/16/08.
3. This excerpt was taken from a longer essay on Winstone Zulu by Mannasseh Phiri accessed at http://oraclesyndicate.twoday.net/stories/3730077/ 9/29/2007. His story is also eloquently told by Stephanie Nolen in her 2007 book *28 Stories of AIDS in Africa*. Portobello Books, London.
4. This quote was taken from a posting on the aidsmythexposed newsgroup. The posting was written by Christine Maggiore in a stream that started 10/18/2007. Accessed at http://www.aidstruth.org/aids-denialists-who-have-died.php.
5. Excerpts taken from the list of denialists who have died posted at AIDSTruth group. An updated list is available at http://www.aidstruth.org/aids-denialists-who-have-died.php.
6. Useful criteria for evaluating health information on the Internet can be found at www.library.cornell.edu/okuref/research/webeval.html and www.quackwatch.com.
7. AIDSTruth.org mission statement available at http://www.aidstruth.org/aids-denialists-who-have-died.php.

Index

Printed in the United States of America